D0463995

Home Remedies
for
Common Ailments

Home Remedies
for Common Ailments

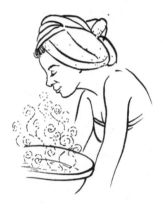

A Handbook of Treatments
for all the Family

Dr James Le Fanu

Robinson
IN COLLABORATION WITH
THE DAILY TELEGRAPH

Robinson Publishing Ltd
7 Kensington Church Court
London W8 4SP

First published by Robinson Publishing Ltd 1997
Reprinted 1997
Copyright © James Le Fanu 1997

A copy of the British Library Cataloguing in Publication Data
for this title is available from the British Library.
ISBN 1–8547–911–1

Important Note
This book is not intended to be a substitute for medical advice
or treatment. Any person with a condition requiring medical
attention should consult a qualified medical practitioner or
suitable therapist.

Printed and bound in Great Britain

Contents

Introduction

The readers of this book will find they will save a lot of time that might otherwise be spent hanging around in the doctor's surgery or casualty department waiting to be seen. They could also save a lot of money that would otherwise be spent on costly pills or medicines from their local chemist for, as will become clear, many minor ailments can be treated more easily and indeed more effectively by remedies readily available in every home. But most important of all, readers will save themselves a lot of unnecessary anxiety by learning what to do when they (or their children) fall victim to the hazards of everyday life – coughs and colds, sore throats, cuts, bruises, boils, skin infections and much else besides.

There is nothing cranky or difficult about the remedies in this book. Rather, they are based on a few quite elementary principles which, once grasped, make them little more than common sense.

In the past many of these simple remedies were common knowledge – but no longer. The remarkable success of modern medicine in the post-war years is mainly to blame in encouraging people to believe they always need doctors with their potent cures to put them right, rather than relying on self-treatment.

This point is perhaps best illustrated by describing the origins of this book. It arose almost by accident from the link made by several readers of two items that appeared in my weekly *Daily Telegraph* column. The first piece described how an inquiry in an American medical journal for advice on a sticky problem: 'a four year old boy had his eyelashes plastered with chewing gum and his mother was unable to remove it. Can you suggest any treatment?' had produced the reply, 'the only remedy appears to be to cut the eyelashes. Most solvents are too toxic for application about the eye.' However, several months later a South African doctor wrote in with an altogether better solution. From his own experience he had noticed that 'if one chews gum while eating milk chocolate, the gum dissolves.' Following this lead, he went on, 'I have repeatedly removed chewing gum from hair by rubbing in soft melted milk chocolate and allowing it to dry. After this the hair is washed well, and the chocolate and the gum come away easily.'

The second piece concerned the effectiveness of the antiviral drug Acyclovir in the treatment of cold sores caused by the herpes virus. Acyclovir is usually prescribed by the family doctor or can now be purchased directly from the chemist for a little over £5. It has, over the years, made a lot of money for the drug company Wellcome who manufacture it. In my column I drew attention to the observations of Graham Worrall, Professor of Medicine, who pointed out that 'systematic review of the evidence shows that Acyclovir is not efficacious in the acute phase of an attack . . . and that it is hardly any better when used prophylactically (as a preventive measure).'

This particular column generated more than the usual amount of correspondence from readers who, it seemed, had fused the message of these two items. Many people reported that they too had found Acyclovir to be 'less than efficacious', in contrast to a variety of little known home remedies including aftershave, whisky, vinegar, and most unusual of all, earwax. These remedies, they claimed, offered a simple solution to the distress caused by recurrent cold sores in the same way that melted chocolate was a simple and effective remedy for hair that had become matted with chewing gum.

Intrigued, I undertook a bit of research – which will be mentioned later – which revealed that there were good scientific reasons why these home remedies should be effective.

When I mentioned these interesting cold sore remedies the following week, the floodgates opened and over the next few months readers kindly sent in an enormous number of home remedies which, in their personal experience, they had found to work for a bewildering variety of different ailments and conditions.

Sorting through these letters it rapidly became clear that there was a lot more to them than simply a collection of 'old wives' tales' that had long been superseded by the onward march of medical progress. Rather, taken together, they added up to a significant body of popular wisdom that had been neglected for too long.

Most of these remedies, not surprisingly, were suggested by people in their seventies or older who had grown up between the wars, before the great medical revolution of the post-war years, when the number of medically effective drugs could almost be counted on the fingers of one hand. Much medical advice at this time was limited to advising on the use of simple remedies which though not necessarily curative could, at least, relieve or diminish symptoms in the hope that eventually they would, with nature's help, get better of their own accord. In their own way these simple remedies – which are the ones we will come across in this book – were actually quite effective. They are no longer recommended by doctors either because they do not know about them or because they believe modern pharmaceuticals are more potent.

Further, the Depression that dominated the inter-war years meant that people could not afford to visit the doctor or buy medicines from the chemist and so they had no alternative but to care for themselves. As one woman described it, 'There was always the feeling that if you went to the doctor you would first be thinking how much money he would want. You would pay for the consultation there and then at the surgery and then after that he would say that if you went round the back, the pharmacist would give you a bottle of medicine. This could work out at 1s 6d (7p) for the visit and 2s 6d (15p) for the medicine and if you didn't have it, well you just waited until you got some money ... or you just did not go to the doctor.'

When medicine had little to offer and people could not afford to go to the doctor, a common-sensical approach to minor ailments was at a premium and it would not be surprising that the reason for the popularity of many of the remedies was quite simply that to a greater or lesser degree they were actually quite effective. They may indeed, as will be seen, work better or at least as well as some pharmaceuticals of the modern age and are certainly less likely to be complicated by side effects. Their wider use would also make people less dependent on medical expertise and more self-confident, and this must be a good thing.

The scientific and other evidence for the efficacy of the remedies described in this book is examined in the next chapter and I will close this introduction on a personal note. I have been a qualified doctor for just over twenty years, the last ten of which have been spent in general practice. I have always been a great believer in the power and scope of modern medicine but while compiling this book I have noticed a significant change in emphasis in the way in which I practise medicine. Now, when someone comes to see me, I naturally reflect on whether or not one or other of the home remedies might be appropriate. I might thus prescribe the 'cold towel treatment' for someone with a sore throat rather than antibiotics, recommend chicken soup rather than cough medicines for bronchitis, or ice cubes rather than steroid ointments for piles.

I was initially apprehensive that patients might be hostile to the suggestion that they might try one or other of these 'old fashioned' remedies rather than being given, as expected, a prescription to take across the road to the pharmacist. But, much to my surprise, this has not been the reaction, rather many are quite happy 'to give it a try'. In a curious way I feel I have exchanged a rather mechanical style of medicine – 'what's wrong, write a prescription, out of the door, next one please', with something richer, almost more profound – 'old fashioned' advice certainly, but also wise and commonsensical and which gives power back to the patient, so the next time round they will not have to seek my advice but know how to treat themselves.

Were this notion of self-treatment to catch on widely, the economic implications would be phenomenal. The conditions described in this book probably account for 70–80 per cent of everyday minor ailments for which the public either seeks medical advice or buys one or other of the over-priced proprietary preparations from the chemist. The potential saving on the nation's drug bill would almost certainly run into hundreds of millions of pounds.

Since preparing this book for press I have continued to receive letters with suggestions and details of recommended home treatments – if you have a favourite remedy I would be most interested to hear about it, and possibly include it in an expanded future edition.

The Evidence

There are two good reasons for being sceptical about the efficacy of self-treatment remedies. The first is the perhaps natural assumption that there is no good scientific evidence that they work – certainly when compared with modern pharmaceuticals which have been rigorously tested. Second, some remedies seem a touch bizarre, so that it is difficult to appreciate what possible justification there could be for their use.

Neither grounds for scepticism is justified as I will show in this chapter. There is much more reliable evidence than might be expected for many of the remedies, while the efficacy of the 'bizarre' turn out, on careful scrutiny, to have quite a simple explanation. This is well illustrated by the three types of remedy for cold sores mentioned in the previous chapter – aftershave, coffee granules and earwax.

The herpes virus responsible for cold sores needs a high humidity to be infective and capable of multiplication – so if the water content in tissues sinks below a certain level, the virus becomes inactivated. The main ingredients of both aftershave (alcohol) and coffee (caffeine) have an astringent effect on tissues, reducing their water content, thus inactivating the virus and promoting healing of the cold sore. Earwax works in a different way altogether. The ear, as a dark moist place, should be an ideal place for infections of all sorts but these are fairly infrequent because earwax contains chemicals inimicable to the proliferation of bacteria, fungi and viruses, including the herpes virus. Further, earwax applied to a cold sore is the perfect material to protect it against exposure to the elements and thus promote healing.

It is possible to identify a similar sensible rationale for virtually all the remedies in this book which turn out to fall into three broad categories. The first category is water, whose main therapeutic properties lie in the physical effects of heat, cold and steam on tissues. The second is food and drink, particularly alcohol. Here again it is the physical and chemical properties that are important. It is necessary to note that, with a few exceptions, this concept of the therapeutic potential of food and drink is quite different from the claims of practitioners of 'alternative medicine' – that certain types of food might cure specific illnesses in the same way that drugs do – that, for example, basil or fennel might cure migraine in the same way as aspirin. This distinction will become obvious. The third category covers the body's own secretions – one of which, earwax, has already been mentioned but also includes saliva and urine.

Water

Water is a chemical miracle and a biological mystery, easily the most complex of all familiar substances. Its composition seems simple enough – two hydrogen atoms flanking one of oxygen – and yet there is no simple explanation for its many peculiar properties. In the gaseous state, whether as steam or water vapour, water molecules are highly independent of each other. Yet in the solid state, as ice, water molecules interact with one

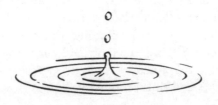

another strongly enough to form an ordered structural lattice. Water is also an excellent, indeed probably the best, solvent within which all chemical compounds have a finite solubility. The many therapeutic possibilities of water depend on the effects its several different forms have on injured and inflamed tissues.

To start with, the human body is 70 per cent water, so the health of tissues is completely dependent on the conservation of water which takes place at two sites – the large bowel and the kidneys. This explains two of its simplest therapeutic uses – in constipation and cystitis.

The main feature of constipation is a hard pellety stool that is difficult to pass, and the easiest way to overcome this is to liquefy the stool by drinking water in quantities greater than the ability of the colon to reabsorb it. 'I became very constipated when pregnant with my first child in 1956' writes Mrs Barbara Willett from Cornwall. 'My family doctor advised "on waking every morning drink half to a pint of warm water . . ." this has worked for me all my life . . . I am seventy-five now and continue to find it infallible'.

The pain and discomfort of cystitis is caused by bacteria inflaming the tissues of the wall of the bladder. The logical solution is to flush the bladder out by drinking sufficient water to overcome the ability of the kidneys to conserve it and thus increase the flow of urine.

Water is an excellent medium for transmitting heat and the next group of water mediated therapies exploits the effect of heat on tissues. When applied directly to the skin, heat dilates the blood vessels thus increasing the blood flow and with it the white blood cells that combat infection. This explains the usefulness of hot compresses when applied to styes or boils which have the effect of bringing these conditions 'to a head' so that they will discharge their infected contents onto the surface of the skin.

When heat penetrates beneath the skin it relaxes muscles that are in spasm, and so hot baths and hot water bottles placed directly on the site of inflamed muscles and joints are particularly popular with arthritis sufferers. In addition, hot wax treatments provide wonderful relief for painful and swollen joints in the hands.

Everything is soluble in water and this includes the crusty nasal secretions which are dissolved by steam inhalation – best achieved by filling a shallow pan with boiling water, placing a towel over the head and inhaling. The efficacy of this treatment has been confirmed in a study conducted by Dr David Tyrrell, director of Medical Research Council's Common Cold Unit as reported in the *British Medical Journal*. Dr Tyrrell showed that the severity of symptoms of cold sufferers was halved in those who regularly used steam inhalation. Along with the direct physical effect of the steam dissolving nasal secretions, Dr Tyrrell commented that the temperature of the steam might also be therapeutically beneficial by modifying the inflammatory response of the nasal tissues to the infecting virus.

Water is also a good medium for transmitting cold, whether in the form of cold baths, ice cubes or a towel wrung out in cold water. This predictably has the reverse effect of heat. It constricts the blood vessels, thus reducing the amount of fluid that leaks out of them.

At the turn of the century cold baths – otherwise known as hydrotherapy – were very popular as treatments for a wide variety of illnesses including typhoid fever, nervous disorders and even tuberculosis. More recently Vijay Kakkar, Professor of Surgical Sciences at London's St Mary's Hospital has investigated the physiological effects of cold baths on the human organism and discovered that amongst other things it boosts the levels of the male and female sex hormones, increases the number of white blood cells that combat infection as well as a naturally occurring blood thinning chemical, TPA, which prevents the blood from clotting, thus reducing the risks of strokes and heart attacks.

Cold – in the form of ice cubes – is particularly effective in relieving the symptoms of piles. Piles are caused by the prolapse of veins around the anal canal which are then pinched tight by the muscles of the anal sphincter, resulting in bleeding and intense pain. Sufferers are advised to sit naked on a chair on which ice cubes have been placed (or a packet of peas from the freezer) wrapped in a clean towel. The coldness of the ice cubes reduces the pain while constricting the prolapsed veins, thus reducing the bleeding from the rectum.

Ice is a similarly useful remedy for sprains and acute muscle injuries by reducing the degree of associated swelling. It is also helpful in the treatment of tennis elbow and similar conditions – the skin should first be oiled, after which an icepack should be placed over the elbow for five to ten minutes twice a day.

Cold water is also the definitive treatment for first degree burns. The coldness suppresses the action of the pain fibres in the skin while the constriction of the blood vessels prevents fluid leaking out, thus minimising the extent of blistering.

Cold water is also a well recognised cure for male infertility due to a low sperm count. This treatment was first described by Dr H. A. Davidson forty years ago who was inspired by a curious experiment in which scientists had placed a woolly bag over a ram's scrotum and noticed its sperm count fell rapidly. He suggested to three subfertile men that they should do the opposite and cold sponge their scrotum twice a day with the result that their wives all conceived almost immediately. The rationale for this treatment is quite straightforward. A cool ambient temperature is essential for adequate sperm production which is why the testes are conveniently placed outside the body. Thus, artificially cooling the testes further by cold sponging or placing them in cold water should boost low sperm counts back up to normal levels.

The final therapeutic use of cold water is for the treatment of sore throats. This is indeed difficult to explain, but many people attest to it, including one of my readers, brought up in Lancashire, whose father was a chemist. The family lived over the shop premises so there was an abundance of proprietary treatments readily available, but when it came to sore throats, 'a large handkerchief was wrung out in cold water,' she reports, 'laid around the neck and covered with a woollen scarf on retiring to bed. As far as I can remember it always worked.'

Alcohol

'Alcohol is the most helpful and hygienic of beverages', observed the great French scientist Louis Pasteur. Unfortunately the general medical antipathy to this 'hygienic beverage' has meant that its medicinal properties have been sadly neglected. Structurally alcohol appears to be very similar to water, the only difference being that one of the hydrogen atoms is replaced by a hydrocarbon. But this small difference opens up a whole vista of therapeutic possibilities both when alcohol is ingested but also when it is applied externally to the skin.

Alcohol's capacity to minimise and suppress the distress of cold sores has already been mentioned but, in general, it is an excellent cleansing agent and antiseptic, and in the form of surgical spirit has been endorsed as an excellent treatment for athlete's foot. Mrs Evelyn Woodfield from Devon writes that she cured her athlete's foot many years ago by using surgical spirit to dab between the toes. She reports that the old skin simply slides away, and the skin beneath is healthy and pink.

Alcohol – in the form of beer – is recommended by hairdressers as a conditioner for dry hair. The suggested technique is to spray the beer on the hair after it has been shampooed and towel dried, but before it is blow dried. The smell of the beer rapidly disperses. Beer can also relieve the symptoms of constipation for the same reason as water, in that it increases the amount of fluid in the bowel, thus liquefying the stool. This effect is compounded by its sugar content which holds on to the water, thus preventing it from being reabsorbed by the colon.

The most distinctive therapeutic use of alcohol arises from its effect, when ingested, on the brain, nerves and the muscles. It provides almost instant relief from the disabling condition of essential tremor and a small dose is an excellent antidote for muscular aches and pains around the shoulders. Alcohol inhibits muscular spasm in the wall of the gut and has been recommended as probably the only effective treatment for infant colic.

Alcohol can also be beneficial for breast-feeding mothers (see pages 31–2).

Food

We eat to live, but food in all its abundance and diversity has always been recognised as having quite specific therapeutic powers. It is beyond the scope of this book to consider or evaluate (if it were possible) the many claims by herbalists and practitioners of natural medicine that the right sort of food can cure each and every ailment. Rather, the food that is described in this section – honey, yoghurt, chicken soup and much else besides – have specific chemical properties which provide a logical rationale for their use in many different conditions.

HONEY

Honey has been valued as a medicinal remedy from the time of the Egyptians primarily because of its healing properties and indeed there is a prescription for a wound salve from an Egyptian papyrus of 2000 BC which includes a mixture of grease, honey and fibre.

Honey is of great value in the treatment of burns and ulcers for two reasons. Firstly, it is more effective at inhibiting the growth of bacteria and other micro-organisms than many commonly used antibiotics. Secondly, honey is very viscous and contains the enzyme catalase which enables it to absorb water from inflamed tissues, keeping wounds clean and preventing further infection.

Dr Robert Blomfield from Chelsea observes:

'I have been using pure natural honey for the past few months in the accident and emergency department where I work and find that applied every two or three days under a dry dressing, it promotes the healing of ulcers and burns better than any other application I have ever used. It can also be readily applied to surface wounds, cuts and abrasions and I can recommend it as a very inexpensive and valuable cleansing and healing agent.'

These sentiments are echoed by Dr A. Zumla of London's Royal Postgraduate Medical School writing in the *Journal of the Royal Society of Medicine*: 'The therapeutic potential of pure uncontaminated honey is grossly undervalued. It is widely available . . . the time has come for conventional medicine to give it its due recognition.'

SUGAR

Sugar has similar wound healing properties to honey. In addition, a teaspoonful dissolved in water in a baby's bottle relieves constipation. It has also recently been noted to be an analgesic and when given to babies prior to having their heels pricked for a blood sample it 'significantly reduces' the amount of crying following the procedure.

SALT

Common salt is the most important source of sodium which is essential for all living cells. In the thousands of years before the invention of refrigeration, salt was the main method of preserving food as it destroys bacteria thus preventing food from going off. This antibacterial effect also explains its function as a local antiseptic. Gargling with warm salt water is the best treatment for infected gums and also useful to reduce the pain of a sore throat. Inhalation up the nose of salt dissolved in water is a standard treatment for children's stuffy noses. Adding a good handful of salt to a bidet or shallow bath and swishing around in the brine provides much relief from the itchiness and discomfort of vaginal thrush.

BICARBONATE OF SODA

Bicarbonate of soda, or sodium bicarbonate, is a granular salt soluble in water. It is an important source of carbon dioxide and is a major component of baking powder and of effervescent beverages such as soda water. Bicarbonate of soda is also an alkali and helps to relieve the burning and discomfort of gastritis caused by excess acidity in the stomach. The burning sensation of cystitis is due to acidity of the urine and this, too, can be minimised by alkalinising the urine with one and a half teaspoonfuls of bicarbonate of soda in water.

Yoghurt

Yoghurt contains the harmless friendly bug lactobacillus that helps suppress the proliferation of the fungal infection candida in the vagina. It is advised that a pint of live yoghurt eaten each day will control the irritation of vaginal thrush, or a small amount on the tip of a tampon can be introduced directly into the vagina.

Chicken Soup

Chicken soup is also known as Jewish penicillin because of the conviction of Jewish mothers that it relieves coughs, colds and other infections of the respiratory tract. In 1849 the Reverend Edmund Dixon recommended cock broth as a cure for coughs. The recipe he favoured involved running an old cock 'till he fall with weariness, then kill and pluck him and boil him until all the flesh falls off, then strain. This broth mollifies . . . and moves the belly'.

Almost 150 years later Dr Kumar Sakethoo of New York's Mount Sinai Medical Center discovered that the beneficial ingredient of chicken soup was a sulphur compound. This increases the velocity of nasal secretions, thus minimising the contact between viruses and the lining of the nose. This explains its usefulness in the treatment of infections of the upper respiratory tract.

FRUIT AND VEG

Fruit and vegetables are an important source of indigestible cellulose that bulks out the content of the stool, thus relieving constipation. Prunes are also a potent laxative and here the vital ingredient is magnesium sulphate. Some people find that cashew nuts are equally effective as a laxative (see page 51).

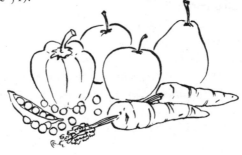

FRUIT JUICE

The juice of the apple and cranberry fruit have anti-infective properties. Apple juice is recommended by Yvonne Wilson from London for the infection of the eyelids known as blepharitis. She suggests peeling off a two inch slice of apple, bending it in half with the skin sides together until the juice appears, then placing gently on the eyelids.

There is substantial evidence that the products of cranberry juice prevent bacteria sticking to the wall of the bladder making it a useful adjunct in the treatment of cystitis. Dr A. E. Sobota from Ohio comments: 'The potential use of cranberry juice in the treatment of urinary tract infections might be particularly beneficial for those who suffer recurrent attacks.'

TEA AND COFFEE

The value of coffee in the treatment of cold sores has already been described, and tea has also been reported as being effective for similar reasons. Tea has other functions as well, including the treatment of blistering after minor burns. Wet teabags should be applied until the pain has been reduced. 'It is, of course, the tannic acid in the tea that is effective' reports Mr G. V. Pride from Dorset. In addition, strained tea has been suggested as an excellent antidote for eye strain.

Coffee contains the chemical methylxanthine, which dilates the airways and this can relieve the symptoms of asthma. In a study of ten patients Dr Schmule Kivity of the Tel Aviv Medical Centre reports that caffeine both improves the performance of lung function and prevented the constriction of the airways.

A FEW CURIOSITIES

Finally, there are a few examples where the efficacy of certain foods in relieving the symptoms of illness can best be described as inexplicable. These include the alleged benefits of lettuce in the relief of insomnia and that avoiding lettuce may reduce the pain of sciatica. Mr J. C. Beard, a retired dentist from Woodford, was surprised to find that his postman's suggestion that he should keep a nutmeg in his hip pocket for the relief of backache, actually worked. And it is claimed that warts can be made to disappear by rubbing them with the inside of a broad bean pod.

Household Items

Besides fulfilling their intended function, several household items to be found in every home can also double up as useful home remedies.

SUPERGLUE

Splitting of the skin at the tips of the fingers or around the heel causes painful fissures which are colloquially known as 'hacks'. Dr J. C. Clarke from Belfast has found these can be rendered instantly painless by the application of superglue, while Mr David Fairburn from Argyle has found that Sellotape is equally beneficial.

TAPE

Tape has been recommended for two different conditions. Applied directly over the patella, it helps relieve the pain of arthritis of the knees, while strong strapping of the chest markedly reduces the discomfort associated with a broken rib.

SURGICAL SPIRIT

The two main uses of surgical spirit as a home remedy have already been noted: applied to the lips in the early tingling stage, it will stop an incipient cold sore and applied between the toes it will cure the most intractable case of athlete's foot.

HAIRDRYER

Hairdryers have two potential uses as home remedies. Firstly, hot air can be soothing when applied to inflamed tissues or joints, so hairdryers may be helpful in relieving the pain of arthritis or following wasp or insect stings. Hairdryers play an important role in the treatment of severe itchiness of the anal canal and vaginal region known respectively as pruritus ani and pruritus vulvae. Dry rubbing with a towel after bathing can exacerbate itchiness in these regions, and using the hot air from a hairdryer is a much better option.

Vaseline

Although there is a jar of Vaseline (petroleum jelly) in every home, its full potential as a home remedy may not be appreciated. Vaseline when applied to the inner surface of the nostrils during and after a heavy cold prevent them from becoming sore and chapped. A vaseline smeared cottonbud gently rotated around the inner surface of the anus relieves the pain of piles and smooths the passage of the stool.

Finally, Vaseline can be used as a preventive measure against cold sores 'brought out' by exposure to sun and wind. Cover the lips with Vaseline and a trip to the beach or a day out sailing can be enjoyed without the fear that a cold sore will erupt the following day.

Autotherapy

The therapeutic value of the body's natural secretions – autotherapy – is at once the most readily available and also the least appreciated of home remedies. The principle is simple. Saliva, urine and earwax all contain chemicals that are inimicable to bacteria and other organisms thus protecting against infections of the mouth, urinary tract and ear respectively. The essence of autotherapy is simply to make use of this property of secretions to treat infection and promote healing.

SALIVA

Those afflicted by the misfortune of a dry mouth not only find it difficult to masticate and digest their food but are particularly prone to recurrent infections of the mouth and gum. Clearly then saliva must contain compounds inimicable to the growth of bacteria including lysozyme that attacks the cell walls of bacteria and lactoferrin that mops up iron necessary for its growth. Other compounds present in saliva prevent bacteria sticking to the side of the mouth or prompt them to come together, enabling them to be swept from the oral cavity by swallowing or spitting. These chemicals are all present in highest concentrations on waking, so, when used as a home remedy, early morning saliva or 'fasting spittle' is particularly recommended.

Saliva can be used to treat styes and to prevent boils erupting. 'Whenever I have an incipient boil – one knows from the feel of it whether it is going to be a boil or just a spot – I apply saliva and after a couple of days it has gone' reports Mr Bryan Evers from West Middlesex. Saliva applied to cuts and abrasions cleanses them and promotes healing – presumably explaining the origin of the term 'kiss it better'.

Mr K. S. M. Sears from Surbiton reports that saliva can help to disperse warts, 'I first discovered this remedy by nibbling away at a wart on the knuckle of one of my fingers', he reports. After a heavy cold the regular application of saliva on the inside of the nostrils will prevent the skin from becoming chapped and painful.

It has been suggested that animal saliva – particularly that of dogs – is even more effective than the human variety. Certainly when a dog is unable, for any reason, to lick its wounds, they tend to fester. The healing potential of canine saliva crops up in the Bible (St Luke 16: 20–1) when Lazarus was waiting at the rich man's gate to be fed with the crumbs which fell from the table, 'the dogs came and licked his sores'.

EARWAX

The earhole being a damp and moist place should be an ideal breeding ground for bacteria and fungi of all sorts. In fact infections of the outer ear – known as otitis externa – are quite rare because earwax, like saliva, contains chemicals that in one way or another inhibit the growth or micro-organisms.

The only therapeutic use of earwax (there may be others) mentioned in this collection is for the treatment of cold sores (page 45). It is interesting to note that the suggestion came (second hand) from a sailor, as cold sores are an occupational hazard of sailors being stimulated by exposure of the skin to the elements – particularly sun, wind and salt water.

URINE

Urine is 95 per cent water, the remaining 5 per cent being made up of mineral salts, hormones and the important chemical urea that accounts for its therapeutic properties. Urine is sterile and so any reluctance to use it as a home remedy is for aesthetic rather than scientific reasons.

Urine therapy is very popular in India where conferences devoted to its many different aspects are organised every year by the Water of Life Foundation. Former Prime Minister Mr Desai famously drank his urine every morning and, though many beneficial results are claimed from this practice, urine therapy in this book is limited to its external applications in the treatment of infection and skin conditions.

The urea present in urine is formed from the breakdown of nitrogen compound. It is an emollient which traps water in the skin and accordingly urea is an important component of several remedies for the treatment of eczema and other skin conditions. Exposure to bricks and mortar is a particularly potent cause of occupational eczema of the hand and bricklayers in particular are aware of urine's valuable properties. 'When old houses built with lime mortar were demolished, it was economical to pay a pensioner to "dress" the bricks for reuse by chipping away the mortar. This made the man's hands very sore, and relief was obtained by urinating on them.' The emollient effect of fresh urine also explains why nursing mothers in the past would wipe their baby's faces with their wet nappies in the hope of improving their complexion.

In his book *The Complete Guide to Urine Therapy*, Mr Coen van der Kroon recommends a urine massage for the treatment of eczema and other simple skin disorders. He favours urine a few days old and notes that its effect is enhanced if heated. 'An entire body massage with urine can take 20 minutes,' he writes, 'allow at least an hour for the urine to be absorbed – afterwards wash off with luke warm water.'

It is well recognised that patients with poor kidney function are susceptible to infections of the urinary tract so clearly a healthy flow of urine must contain chemicals inimicable to the proliferation of bacteria. The anti-infective properties of urine have been investigated by Dr J. U. Shlegel of the Tulaine University School of Medicine in New Orleans who found that urea present in similar concentrations to that found in urine was highly effective against four separate groups of bacteria. This provides a theoretical rationale for treating, as recommended by Mr van der Kroon, conjunctivitis and ear infections with a few drops of urine or, more contentiously, gargling with urine as an antidote to gum infections and a sore throat.

Finally, Dr Amanda Adler of the University of Washington describes an unusual but highly efficacious use of urine as a home remedy in the prevention of frostbite. 'While leaving school with a temperature of thirty-five degrees Fahrenheit below zero, a young Alaskan boy stopped to lick a handrail and was immediately frozen to it by his tongue and lip. His father attempted to free him but could not, so instead he urinated into the boy's mouth.' This it seems did the trick and Dr Adler commends this first aid technique to any quick thinking bystanders who may find themselves in a similar situation.

HAIR

There are two circumstances in which hair can be used as a home remedy. The first is to remove grit from the eye, where a small noose of hair can be used to flick out the offending foreign object without fear of damaging the cornea. Hair also counteracts the exquisite pain and copious tears in those who accidentally rub their eye after touching a chilli – as described by Dr Richard Roberts, a geneticist from Texas. He once experienced these symptoms when in the company of several Mexican friends who urged him to put hair in the affected eye immediately. Though incredulous he tried this and the pain and tears cleared immediately.

Conclusion

The most striking thing to emerge from this chapter is the extraordinary scope of home remedies – indeed it is hard to imagine an everyday hazard or illness which is not treatable in one way or another without the need to visit the doctor or pay good money to the pharmacist.

The range of remedies is so comprehensive it might seem difficult to remember them all, but this can be made a lot easier by thinking about them in relation to the functions of different rooms in every house. Start in the kitchen, whose ready supply of running water is the basis of many treatments – cold water for burns, hot water for stings, ice from the fridge for piles and muscular aches and pains, boiling water from the kettle for coughs and colds. In the fridge can be found live yoghurt for the treatment of thrush, chicken soup waiting to be warmed up for bronchial conditions, and cream for the treatment of heartburn. In the food and vegetable rack are apples for blepharitis, potatoes for burns, and in the pantry cupboard, tea, coffee, salt, bicarbonate of soda, olive oil, vinegar and honey – all of which have distinct therapeutic properties. Next door in the utility room there will be a small tube of superglue and a roll of Sellotape for treating 'hacks' and a bottle of surgical spirit for athlete's foot.

Upstairs in the bathroom there is more water, this time in the form of hot and cold baths for the treatment of aching bones and joints, a bidet full of salt for minor attacks of thrush. Here too is the hairdryer so useful for those with an itchy bottom, and the jar of Vaseline with its multiplicity of functions. The bathroom is also the place where those so inclined might wish to test out the potential of urine therapy.

So home remedies are not quaint old wives'

tales. Rather, as this chapter demonstrates, virtually all have their own logical rationale and are
nothing more than the application of
commonsensical solutions to simple problems.

Acne

Acne is the great physical misfortune of teenage years which can, when severe, cause extensive scarring of the face. Luckily, this can now be avoided by a judicious combination of antibiotics, either taken by mouth or applied directly to the skin, and the potent drug tretinoin.

It is probably fair to say these treatments are overused, especially in milder cases, and in general it would seem undesirable – as often happens – that young people should take antibiotics for a year or even longer.

To appreciate the role of other remedies it is necessary to encapsulate what is believed to cause acne. Essentially the rising levels of testosterone around puberty increases the production of oily sebum by little glands associated with the hair follicles on the face. The cells lining the follicles can form a plug behind which this sebum accumulates which may then be infected by bacteria resulting in the typical spots. Antibiotics attack the infection while cleansing preparations bought directly from the chemist such as benzoyl peroxide cause the plug of cells in the hair follicle to disintegrate thus releasing the blocked infected sebum behind.

The following suggestions may also be useful.

Diet: It is commonly believed that several foods, in particular chocolate and fish, can exacerbate acne and so are best avoided. It is difficult to be certain of the validity of this advice but Mrs K. R. Smith from Bedford describes the benefits of dietary manipulation for her daughter's acne:

> 'My daughter had very bad acne before anyone else of her age. After several years of antibiotics and creams and 'you'll grow out of it' from her

doctor I took her to a homeopath. She changed her diet – no milk products or orange juice mainly – took her off the antibiotics and the result was amazing. She still had a few spots but her skin has been better ever since.'

Clean the skin: Thorough cleansing of the skin will both cut down the number of bacteria and keep the hair follicles open as Mr H. J. Allen reports from his experience with a loofah:

'When I was a teenager my friend and workmate suffered severely with acne and his face was a mass of spots and sores. The doctor advised him to use a 'loofah' instead of a flannel to wash his face. My friend did not know what a loofah was so the doctor went to his bathroom and brought one out to show him. A loofah is the fibrous part of the dried teapod of the luffa, a species of gourd. Using the loofah has a scrubbing effect and is rather painful at first but the important thing is that it stimulates the circulation and helps to remove impurities. My friend's spots cleared in a matter of weeks. I, too, used a loofah although my spots were few. Over the years I have passed on this advice to a number of young people.'

Avoid oil based cosmetics: This seems sensible enough as a lot of oil on the skin will encourage acne formation.

Squeeze the spot: It is not a good idea to squeeze pimples or whiteheads, but where there is a head of pus at the centre of the acne spot or a blackhead, they will heal much more quickly once they are popped. Here the gold wedding ring remedy comes in handy as described by Mrs Mary Goodby from Cheshire.

'Hold ring very firmly by its edge between finger and thumb and very slowly draw the edge of it over the chin, sides of nose and forehead with a very gentle pressure on the skin in a sort of slow motion sweeping or scraping action. Dozens of surprised blackheads and spots will pop out. The secret is to move the ring so firmly and slowly (although gently) that it hardly seems to be moving. Wash the ring and dry it well after each sweeping movement as it will be disgustingly gunged up. The pores will now look a bit odd, like lots of tiny holes, but will soon close up. Repeat every two weeks to keep teenagers' acne at bay.'

Arthritis

Modern medical treatments for arthritis are thankfully very effective both in minimising the acute symptoms of pain and swelling, preventing the progressive damage to joints, and most dramatically of all, replacing damaged joints altogether. None, however, are completely effective, and patients will always have a degree of pain and discomfort from their symptoms for which there are probably more home remedies than for any other condition. These range from copper bracelets and bee stings to thrashing the affected joints with nettles. Some of the following home remedies will be well known to those with arthritis but those that are not are well worth a try.

Heat: Hot or warm baths twice a day are life saving for many of those with arthritis. A jacuzzi is even better for those that can afford it and if they cannot there is always the option of paying a visit to the local health club.

Ice: Sprains and other acute injuries of the muscle

are best treated with an ice pack (or packet of frozen peas) wrapped in a towel and applied directly. Heat is an inappropriate remedy here as it encourages the release of fluid from the damaged muscles which then increases the size of the swollen area dramatically. Ice packs are also an appropriate remedy for tennis elbow and similar conditions as described by Judy Swaine, physiotherapist from Essex: 'Oil the skin and place an ice pack over the elbow for five to ten minutes, twice a day. Rest the arm but ensure you can fully straighten the elbow twice a day. If still very painful after seventy-two hours seek further medical help.'

Towels: This remedy is very similar to that recommended for sore throats and here is described by Pauline Caseley from West Sussex. 'First wring out a towel in cold water which should be wrapped around the affected joint and covered with a woollen scarf or garment, not too tightly. This should be fastened securely in place. Then put on your pyjamas and go to bed. A gentle heat will begin to permeate the joint comforting and relieving the pain and swelling. Remove in the morning.'

Tape: The tape remedy as described by Professor Paul Dieppe and colleagues from Bristol may be a useful supplementary treatment along with 'quads' exercises for those with osteoarthritis of the knee: 'The principle is that the malalignment of the patella in the knee joint may cause an abnormal distribution of pressures in the knee which is corrected by placing a tape directly over the patella so that it shifted towards the midline.' Specialist advice from a physiotherapist is probably necessary to learn the precise technique, but afterwards it can be applied regularly at home.

Massage: An instinctive reaction to any ache or

pain is to massage it, thus improving the circulation and bringing warmth to the affected part. Massage, preferably with the aid of essential oils is an excellent treatment, though interestingly the results always seem much better when someone else is doing it.

Wax: Wax treatments provide wonderful relief for painful and swollen joints in the hands. This Do-It-Yourself recipe comes from an excellent book *Arthritis: what really works* by Dava Sobel and Arthur Klein:

> 'Melt a couple of packages of canning paraffin in a tall pot to fill it about half way and then mineral oil should be added until it is three-quarters full and the mixture should be stirred well. Next the pot should be removed from the heat and left to cool until a light skin forms over the paraffin. Then keeping the fingers slightly apart dip one hand and wrist in quickly and out again. The paraffin should be allowed to dry slightly between dips which should be repeated about ten times. The hands should then be covered with a plastic bag and wrapped with a warm towel left on for twenty minutes during which time the hand should be kept still or alternatively hand exercises can be performed in the soothing heat. The paraffin should then be peeled off and saved for use another time. The process should then be repeated on the other hand and when finished the hands and fingers should be massaged with the mineral oil that remains on the skin.'

Diet: Arthritis, like any other condition, may be relieved or exacerbated by certain foods, though which foods are relevant for which individuals can really only be found by trial and error. Fish, particularly oily fish, is thought to be particularly beneficial while the exclusion of dairy foods, toma-

toes and white potatoes from the diet can sometimes bring dramatic relief.

In addition some people find their arthritis
made better or worse by the most unlikely of foods
as the following two accounts illustrate. It is well
worthwhile to be on the lookout for similar situations. Mr Andrew Stronach from Kent suffered
from chronic low back pain and lumbago for a
period of ten years. He had been advised by two
separate specialists that he would need to have an
operation to relieve the pressure on the nerves in
the spinal cords which were responsible for his
symptoms. He noticed on reading *The Times* one
day a reader's letter which claimed that many
people had experienced lumbago as a result of
eating lettuce:

> 'As I had suffered the torture of the damned on
> and off for over ten years I decided to stop eating
> the stuff. No more pain, no more stiffness! A look
> back at the events of the past proved convincing.
> I had first had the problem while on an artillery
> exercise during National Service when, for some
> reason, we had been given lettuce every day for a
> fortnight – rare enough to be memorable. Since
> then I only suffered when living with my wife or
> my mother both of whom always gave me regular
> salads (when living on my own I never bothered).
> Subsequently I have been free of pain except for
> those few occasions when I have succumbed to
> temptation and eaten lettuce. Even a leaf in a
> sandwich can give me the odd twinge the next
> day. The symptoms are definitely not psychoso-
> matic nor am I a believer in alternative medicine.
> I just happened to be lucky enough to have found
> the cause of something that was wrecking my life.
> I wonder how many others are not so lucky.'

Conversely, Mr J. C. Beard, a retired dentist from
Watford reports on a type of food that relieved his
back pain – though this one he did not have to eat:

'I am a retired dental surgeon of the "old fashioned school" who always stooped whilst operating on my patients in an orthodox dental chair. Naturally, I suffered the occasional back ache until a postman patient recommended that I should keep a nutmeg in my hip pocket. Full of scepticism I tried it, and now after thirty years or so I am never without one. I mentioned this to an angling friend and to my surprise he assured me that for many years he had hung a small bag of nutmeg from his bedpost to ward off night cramps! This may be auto-suggestion or witchcraft, but we agreed, as do many of my patients who tried it, that it does work for us.'

Athlete's Foot

Athlete's Foot is caused by a fungus picked up from the swimming pool or communal washroom floor. It gets a hold between the toes where the combination of high humidity and warm temperature encourages the propagation of its spores. Very soon the skin is cracked and macerated which is both painful and very itchy.

The most striking feature of athlete's foot is its intractability – once acquired it will rumble on for years with intermittent acute exacerbations, proving remarkably resilient to the host of antifungal creams prescribed by doctors or purchased over the counter from chemists.

The main reason why athlete's foot fails to respond to antifungal remedies is that after a while the condition is sustained by various types of bacteria that take advantage of the unhealthy tissue between the toes. These in turn are responsible for emitting a variety of foul smelling odours with names like putrescin and cadavarine that are mainly responsible for the unappetising odour that accompanies athlete's foot.

Athlete's foot is thus an ecological wonderland inhabited by both fungi and bacteria which are difficult to eradicate by conventional treatment but respond, often dramatically, to traditional home remedies.

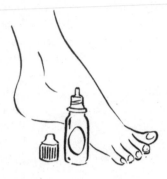

Surgical spirit: 'I cured my athlete's foot over twenty years ago by dabbing surgical spirit between the toes. The old skin slides off, leaving lovely healthy pink skin for ever as long as you keep off the talcum. Thereafter a daily dab of cheap toilet eau de cologne between the toes is all they need.' Mrs Evelyn Woodfield from Devon.

Mr G. D. Adams from Northamptonshire also found that placing the feet in a bowl of surgical spirit, 'the infection sloughed off, leaving the most beautiful pink baby skin behind with no sign of athlete's foot'. In addition he put his socks on while his feet were still wet and sterilised his shoes by sloshing the spirit into them.

Lavender oil: When spending the weekend at a conference, Lady Yardley from Oxford discovered she had left behind her 'rather ineffective anti-athlete's foot cream'. 'I did have some lavender oil with me which I like to use in the bath and which seemed worth trying. I was amazed to find that after a few days the persistent infection had healed completely. Cracks in the flesh were still there – but the skin was healthy.'

Pasteurisation: Mr Basil Gotto from County Cork picked up his athlete's foot in Singapore and found pasteurisation an effective remedy. 'Instead of using hot water, I used cold. After a hot bath I put my foot straight from the hot water to under the cold tap. It works for me every time.'

Ultra violet light: 'In my experience over many years, ultra violet rays are a far more effective remedy than the usual creams and powders. The lamp I use is more than twenty years old (Phillips Ultraphil Special HP3114). It requires only about five minutes exposure of the top and bottom of the toes turning them to allow the light into the affected area for three days in succession. This is less than causes any reddening of the skin,' reports John Shelton from Middlesex.

Miscellaneous: A reader from Winchester recommends 'a small paintbrush dipped in iodine', Mr P. G. Shingler from Hove suggests Friar's balsam; and Mrs Mary Parsons from Devon aloe vera – 'a veritable panacea'.

Boils

When a hair follicle becomes infected by bacteria, pus forms, resulting in a boil – an inflamed lump with a white centre. Boils are usually a trivial condition which resolve once they burst after which the skin heals. Young men, in particular, seem to

Boils

be particularly prone to multiple, painful boils, especially on their neck.

The main value of home remedies is to 'ripen' the boil by bringing it to a head by cupping or applying a poultice.

Cupping: The technique of cupping is described by Jill Nice, author of *Herbal Remedies and Home Comforts*: 'One takes a small-mouthed jar well rinsed in boiling water and as soon as is feasible without scalding the patient the mouth of the jar is placed over the boil until it cools. Suction does the rest and provided the boil is at a stage ready for treatment the core will come out neatly and without unnecessary pain.'

Hot compresses: Hot compresses are the most reliable method of bringing a boil to a head. The simplest technique being to apply cottonwool which has been dipped in hot water to which salt has been added.

Dock leaves: Mr Alan Grant from Devon describes his experience with dock leaves.

> 'Whilst serving with the RAF I contracted four boils on the back of my neck. I was working in the medical section at the time but conventional treatments were not working so in despair I went to the local pub to numb the pain and discomfort. A local farmworker spotted the dressing on my neck and being told I had boils, told me to apply dock leaves. Upon returning to camp I found two large dock leaves and applied them to the affected area, covered with a bandage. The following morning, I removed the bandage and there on the dock leaves were four boils completely drawn out (the fifth was a 'blind' boil which was subsequently lanced).'

Saliva: The anti-infective properties of saliva may prevent a boil developing according to **Mr Bryan Evers** from West Middlesex. 'Whenever I have an incipient boil – one knows from the feel of it after experiencing one whether it is a boil or just a spot – I apply saliva and in a couple of days it has gone. Several friends have cured their boils in the same way – very simple too.'

Breast Feeding

Hundreds of books and articles have been written about breast feeding over the last few years full of practical advice to which there is little to add other than the following observations.

The mother's diet: Maternal breast milk tastes like watered down milk fortified with teaspoonfuls of sugar. If this oversweet liquid was the only taste experience for the newborn, one might expect them to get bored with it fairly quickly. But the flavour of breast milk varies markedly depending on the maternal diet. Many mothers report that their baby's behaviour is strongly influenced by what they themselves have had to eat. Thus the flatus inducing properties of beans and lentils will result in both mother and child passing lots of wind. Similarly, maternal onion eating is said to cause infantile colic, spicy foods and acidic drinks lead to stomach upsets and chocolate notoriously results in diarrhoea.

Alcohol: Alcohol is held to be doubly beneficial. It increases milk production – malt beer is particularly recommended – while its appearance in breast milk is soothing and sleep inducing. There is no evidence that this is harmful in moderation though there is one account of a woman who took the 'alcohol is good for nursing mothers' rather too literally and whose consumption of fifty lagers a week produced signs of chronic alcoholism in her baby.

Cabbage leaves: Raw cabbage leaves applied directly to the surface of the breast are said to reduce the physical discomfort associated with excess milk production. Their shape is peculiarly suited to this function while their coolness is an effective antidote to heat and soreness. This claim is validated by a study conducted by doctors in South Africa who found that women who regularly applied cabbage leaves were more likely to breast feed exclusively and to do so for longer.

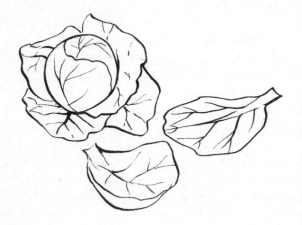

Broken Rib

For obvious reasons those who fall and sustain a broken rib find breathing, and particularly coughing, very painful, as movement of the rib irritates the nerve fibres around the fracture. As with all fractures this can take up to six weeks to resolve and can be complicated by lung infections as pain on coughing makes it difficult to expectorate retained secretions.

Virtually everyone who breaks a rib will end up in casualty where, after an X-ray has been taken to ensure there are not associated injuries such as a collapsed lung, it is customary to send the patient on their way with some painkillers and advice that as the rib heals the pain will diminish.

At one time it was customary to strap the rib with adhesive tape, though this fell out of fashion. Nonetheless, strapping certainly does relieve the pain as Dr K. Norcross of Birmingham's Dudley Road Hospital observes. He analysed the records from the casualty department at Manchester Royal Infirmary before rib strapping fell out of favour. 'In 44 cases, 27 were relieved of pain by strapping, in four it was made worse and 13 gained no relief. Clearly for most patients strapping is effective in the relief of pain – if it is not it can be removed immediately.' He describes the case of one woman he treated: 'She told me she had severe pain from a fracture of the eighth rib and that before strapping was applied every breath had been very painful and she could not cough at all. Within an hour of strapping she was virtually pain-free, could breathe readily and cough and clear her chest. She was most grateful for the help that had been provided.' Dr Norcross describes the technique as follows: 'To be effective strapping must splint the chest on the affected side so it must be applied under moderate tension to the chest in full expiration. The strapping should cross the midline to the nipple in front and scapula at the back. In hairy men, shaving of the chest is needed first. The strapping must be inextensible (i.e. two inch zinc oxide strapping).'

Bruises

Bruises are caused by bleeding of small blood vessels under the skin and so the most appropriate treatment is the same as for bleeding cuts – apply pressure.

> 'I remember my father getting into our car which was one of the fifties Rovers with the front door opening towards the back and the back door opening towards the front leaving a pillar in the middle. He was getting back into the car with his hand on this pillar when someone slammed the other door. He pressed his hand hard for some time as we drove on and had no bruising or swelling at all.' Marion Banyard from Suffolk.

Alternatively, if available, cold ice packs (or frozen peas from the freezer) will both reduce the swelling and bruising from a bump by constricting the blood vessels under the skin thus preventing blood and fluid leaking into the surrounding tissue.

Burns

The intensity of burns are graded to 'first', 'second' and 'third' degree depending on the extent of tissue damage. Second degree burns cause immediate blistering and third degree, where the skin will appear white or charred, require medical attention and so the following remedies should only be used for those with 'first degree' where the skin is reddened and painful.

For historical reasons there is often some confusion about whether the best immediate treatment for burns is cold water or some soothing oily compound such as olive oil or butter. Prior to the Second World War cold water was believed to be dangerous for burns as being more likely to be followed by infection and butter or olive oil were advocated instead. During the War, however, this view was turned on its head and water was found to be highly effective. The belief that oily compounds were valuable clearly persisted – a point well illustrated by Mr S. A. Skinner from Watford:

> 'Over sixty years ago, when I was about ten years old, holidaying on a farm during haymaking I mistakenly leaned on the tractor and put my hand (palm and fingers) on the exhaust manifold. As you can imagine, I received a very severe burn. We set off back to the farmhouse in search of the then treatment – olive oil! Unfortunately none was found and I was in such pain that I put my hand under the cold spring that flowed out of the farmhouse water supply. Each time I withdrew my hand the pain returned so I stayed there most of the afternoon. When I finally took my hand away – maybe after two or three hours – there was no more pain. There were no blisters, no scarring and no after-effects at all. My daughter subsequently became the Sister in Charge of the Regional Burns Unit and it seems that my accidental treatment was about fifty years ahead of its time.'

Cold water is the immediate first aid remedy for burns but contributors have also suggested a variety of other useful agents that can be applied to ease the pain and stinging over the subsequent days until the burn has healed.

Potatoes: Potatoes are the most frequently cited of the food based remedies for burns and can be applied raw, as potato skins or mashed. 'As a child playing at being a blacksmith, I burnt my fingers badly. My mother boiled potatoes, mashed them and wrapped my hands in the mash. They soon healed without any scars.' Mrs Mary King from Suffolk.

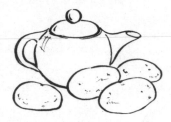

Tea: Tea, too, has its advocates and is easily applied in the form of teabags. 'Used and wet teabags should be applied, being kept moist until the pain has been reduced – being kept on for several hours if necessary. This will often prevent blistering where it would otherwise have occurred. It is, of course, the tannic acid in the tea that is effective.' Mr G. V. Pride from Dorset.

Aloe vera: Aloe vera seems to be a panacea for all ills. Ms J. Orritt from Winchester reports: 'As a sufferer from multiple sclerosis with poor coordination, I am frequently burning or scalding myself but since discovering aloe vera I have no fear as it is guaranteed to work.' Aloe vera may be kept as a plant in the kitchen – when all that is necessary is to break off a leaf and squeeze the moisture onto the affected skin or alternatively it can be obtained in a gel form from most pharmacists or health food shops.

I have heard of two further unusual remedies which are perhaps more difficult to recommend. The first is heat. Blacksmiths and others working with hot metal strongly believe that the best treatment for burns was heat as Mr T. R. Pearce from Middles-brough recalls:

> 'I began my apprenticeship in marine engineer-ing in 1936 and was soon set to work with plumbers. Copper pipes were brazed together but gloves were not worn and burns were frequent. The first time I was careless enough to grasp the hot part of a pipe in error, I was quickly taken to the brazier and my hand held over it for a few minutes until I could no longer bear it.'

The second is nasal secretions. Mr Jeremy Nichols from East Lothian reports an old Suffolk black-smith's somewhat offputting treatment for burns which he learnt while farming in East Anglia:

> 'Following a burn, blow your nose and apply the result on as liberally as possible on the painful area.'

Mr Nichols and his wife say they have benefited from this treatment for the past 25 years, but admit that 'all our medical friends have shown polite interest in our claims but have shown great reluc-tance to try it out for themselves!'.

Chilblains

Chilblains are very itchy, reddish-blue swellings, usually of the hands and feet, induced by cold which restricts the circulation of blood to the extremities (to keep the core warm) thus depriving these tissues of oxygen. They have been relatively rare since the almost universal introduction of central heating but can be a serious nuisance for those with poor circulation.

The following remedies have been suggested:

Chilblains

Urine: 'As a child I suffered in agony from chilblains and I can still remember the pain and itching. One day when the problem was discussed with a lady visitor, she said to my mother "let her stand in her own water". Although I am now in my seventies, I can still remember that moment which banished forever the suffering of chilblains.' Anon.

Other contributors have similar comments. 'I remember an old cobbler in my village quite a few years before the last war when chamber pots were in general use. He used to say there is nothing so good for chilblains as to soak the affected part in your own water.' D. Fryer from Yorkshire.

Soda: 'Back in the 1920s at the onset of every winter, chilblains were one of the commonest ailments in our family. The invaluable remedy was a lighted wax candle and a large piece of washing soda. The soda was held in the flame of the candle until melting-point and the hot liquid applied straight to the affected part. Done in the evening, it resulted in dirty sheets but that was a small price to pay for the relief which usually lasted the winter.' T. W. Palmer from Dorset.

Onion: 'My chilblains would last for months each winter until I tried cutting an onion in half and rubbing the cut edge against the chilblain. Its juice soon got rid of the itching and the severity died down.' Shirley de Ath from Hampshire.

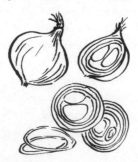

Choking

Choking is a potential catastrophe, and one of those emergency situations where awareness of the appropriate treatment promptly performed can be life saving. The first imperative is to make the correct diagnosis – and particularly to distinguish choking from a heart attack. Here, luckily, there is one vital clue: the victim is silent. The obstructing piece of food as well as preventing air from getting into the lungs, prevents air from passing over the vocal chords, which is necessary for speech. One way to recognise the emergency is to point at the dinner plate and ask 'Can you speak?' If the victim cannot, one can be sure he has food stuck in the throat – and be equally sure he will die in a few minutes unless someone acts fast. The following manoeuvres to dislodge the obstruction are recommended.

Raise the left arm: It is not clear why this should work – but several readers attest to it. The arm should be raised 'as though trying to touch the ceiling – or the sky'.

Remove the obstruction: The common initial reaction is to stick the forefinger or middle finger into the victim's throat in the hope of extracting the bolus of food. This is not a very good idea as, quite apart from the danger of having one's digit severely bitten, it can precipitate a spasm at the back of the throat which only makes matters worse. Nonetheless, if the victim can be encouraged to explore the back of his own throat, it is sometimes possible to get hold of the obstructing matter – particularly if it is a large piece of meat.

Slap on the back: It is a time honoured reaction to thump the victim vigorously on the back. This, too, is unlikely by itself to do much good, though it may stimulate a coughing fit which can disimpact the obstruction. By contrast, back slapping may do the trick in small children if they are also held upside down to benefit from the added effects of gravity.

Heimlich's manoeuvre: The manoeuvre perfected by Henry Heimlich requires a sharp blow in the midline just underneath the diaphragm forcing air out of the lungs under pressure. This mechanism can be simulated by inserting a cork into the mouth of an inflated balloon and squeezing it forcefully. The cork flies out, similar to the opening of a bottle of champagne.

The technique is as follows: stand behind the victim and put both arms around the waist. Make a fist with one hand and place the thumb side against the victim's abdomen just above the navel. Grasp the fist with the other hand and press it forcefully into the abdomen with a quick inward and upward thrust. Repeat five time pausing between each thrust to see if the obstruction has been dislodged.

In the twenty years since Mr Heimlich first described his manoeuvre its efficacy has been confirmed many times. Objects expelled from the throats of choking victims have included apples, hot-dogs, beef, chicken, coins, pills and sweets. One mother found her nine month old infant blue and lifeless in her cot and noticed that foam rubber had been gouged out of the mattress cover. A quick thrust on the baby's abdomen and the missing rubber flew out of the child's throat.

Choking alone: Dr Marilyn Dover, a social scientist from Exeter, has described the experience of choking without anyone to help her. Eating bacon and egg one evening in front of the television, 'I swallowed a morsel of food I had scarcely begun to chew . . . I was not breathing, there was not the tiniest particle of air going into or out of my windpipe', she writes. 'I sat with what felt like a brick in my throat, relatively calmly listing my options and looking for the best solution.' For those choking alone the Heimlich manoeuvre is useless as it cannot be performed on oneself because hitting the abdomen is met with a reflex tightening of the abdominal muscles. Appreciating this Dr Dover performed a variation on this manoeuvre on herself: 'I stood up, placed my clenched fist over my diaphragm [i.e. at the top of the abdomen just below the sternum], bent over double quickly simultaneously squeezing my chest with my elbows to expel the air in my lungs.' At first nothing happened, and she tried again. This time 'the obstruction moved, it suddenly popped out of my mouth'. An alternative technique is to press the upper abdomen quickly over any firm surface such as the back of a chair or edge of table.

Colds

Despite intensive scientific research conducted by the Medical Research Council's Common Cold Unit over many years, a cure for this, the most common of all viral infections, has proved elusive. At one time it was hoped that the expensive anti-viral compound 'interferon' might be of value. Besides being very expensive, it potential as a remedy was finally abandoned when it was found its side effects were the same or even worse than the cold itself – including tiredness, malaise and muscular aches and pains.

There are a host of remedies that, it is claimed, will prevent a cold developing, of which the most famous, promoted by the late Nobel prize-winner, Linus Pauling, is an extra large dose of vitamin C. This selection is, however, restricted to treatment of the main symptom – a stuffy nose.

Steam: Steam inhalation, as the cheapest and most effective of remedies, should be used much more frequently. It is much preferable to the decongestant medications procured at considerable cost from the local chemist. Boiling water is placed in a shallow pan into which a drop of menthol, or eucalyptus oil may be added, and a towel is placed over the head. After 15 minutes of steam inhalation the nostrils will be clear – at least for a while. Some people prefer to go to the bathroom, close the windows, place a towel against the door and sit on the side of the bath inhaling the steam from a really hot bath or shower.

Salt: Mr P. J. Fenerty from Liverpool learned the salt remedy from his grandfather who was born in 1874. One heaped teaspoon of salt is dissolved in a bottle of water and placed in the hollow of the hand and snuffled up the nose. 'It always works better than the proprietary remedies prescribed by the doctor,' comments Mr Fenerty who also enclosed a letter from *The Times* pointing out that in 1919 during the height of the post-war flu epidemic: 'The only people who escaped completely were those who had used salt water constantly.'

Alcohol: Mrs Mirren Coxon passed her pre-1914 childhood in Easter Ross in the north of Scotland where they suffer from a lot of colds. 'My father took charge and stood over us while we swallowed a mug of hot toddy – whisky, honey and hot water. It cured the cold and had the added bonus of putting us off whisky for life.'

Chicken soup: Chicken soup is also known as Jewish penicillin because of a long-standing belief held by Jewish mothers that it relieves infections of the upper respiratory tract. Interestingly, the dietary instructions to Moses on Mount Sinai specifically permitted chicken and some believe the recipe for chicken soup was given to Moses on this occasion. The beneficial ingredient of the soup has recently been identified as a sulphur compound which increases the velocity of nasal secretions by almost a third thus promoting the elimination of the infective viral particles from the nose.

Vaseline: As the cold begins to resolve, the nostril openings may be inflamed and painful from the repeated trauma of nose blowing. Vaseline applied on a cottonwool bud is an effective remedy and saliva is also reputedly useful in preventing crusts and scabs forming around the nostrils.

Cold Sores

Cold sores play an important role in this anthology of remedies because they are responsible for starting the project off. Cold sores are caused by the herpes virus which lurks in the nerves around the mouth. Most of the time they cause no symptoms but periodically they track down a nerve to the surface of the skin where initially they cause a tingling sensation followed by the appearance of one or more blisters. These last several days before scabbing over. An attack may come out of the blue but more usually is precipitated by one or other of several types of stress – including a respiratory infection or exposure of the skin to cold or sunlight.

The standard treatment for the last ten years has been the antiviral drug Acyclovir either in the form of a cream or, for those with severe recurrent attacks, taken in the form of tablets. The best results are obtained when Acyclovir is used at the tingling stage of the attacks, but it is most commonly prescribed once the blisters have already appeared, by which time its efficacy is much less convincing. Professor Graham Worrall, writing in the *British Medical Journal*, maintained that Acyclovir is only of 'marginal benefit'. If the pills are taken regularly it reduces the frequency of episodes in those seriously affected. Several contributors commented that Acyclovir had been of little use and as it is costly – at £5 for a cream and £30 for a course of tablets – their alternative remedies are of great interest.

Alcohol and spirits: Mr F. W. Sanders from Suffolk commended the after shave lotion Tabac Original. 'This does not completely stop the cold sores but is a tremendous boon. The earlier the application, the greater and better the relief.' The active ingredient is almost certainly the alcohol base of the after shave as indeed must be the case with several other recommended remedies, including perfumes, whisky, spirits of camphor, surgical spirit, vinegar and TCP. Dr Svante Travenius explains how alcohol works: 'The herpes virus (that causes the cold sore) needs a high humidity to be effective and capable of multiplication. If the water content in the tissues sinks under a certain minimum, the virus becomes inactivated. Alcohol is a dehydrating agent. This reduces the available water content in the sites affected by the virus, with the result that it is made ineffective and the sores heal.'

Coffee: Caffeine, the main constituent of coffee has been shown to inhibit the herpes virus which may account for the excellent results reported by Mr W. I. Drysdale from Devon: 'When you get that telltale tickle, simply dip your finger into the residue of a cup of instant black coffee and rub on the affected part. The coffee must not be decaffeinated. It need not be unnecessarily strong.' Mr Drysdale reports that fellow sufferers to who he has commended this remedy have been equally impressed but 'when I have mentioned it to a variety of professional people including pharmacists and doctors I have been greeted with a half-closed eye and a suggestion of a smirk'.

Earwax: Sailors are particularly prone to cold sores as the combination of sun and wind is well recognised to be a major precipitating factor, so this suggestion from Mr K. E. Smith from Gwynedd is of particular interest: 'Fifty years ago a sailor (before the mast!) suggested I use my own earwax. Distasteful maybe, but I have never had any trouble since and neither has anyone to whom I have passed on the tip.' The rationale for this remedy is presumably a mixture of the protective effect of the wax and its anti-infective properties.

Vaseline: The opportunity to prevent cold sores emerging is limited but as just noted, exposure to the elements is a frequent precipitant so those prone to recurrent attacks should, when outdoors or on the beach on holiday, make sure they cover their lips with generous doses of Vaseline.

Conjunctivitis

Conjunctivitis, otherwise known as pink eye, can either be caused by an infection – where there will be a greenish discharge or crusting of the eyelids in the morning, or by an allergy – most usually hay fever when itching is a prominent symptom, or by an irritant such as chillies.

INFECTIVE CONJUNCTIVITIS

Standard treatment for infective conjunctivitis is an antibiotic cream or eyedrops, but many cases will clear with simple hygienic measures.

Warm water compresses: Dip a flannel in warm water and apply it to the eye three or four times a day for ten minutes. In addition, a cottonwool bud dipped in a bowl of warm water with a couple of drops of baby shampoo can be used to clear away the crusts from the eyelids.

Apple juice: Apple juice is recommended for blepharitis – infection of the eyelids – which may be associated with conjunctivitis or come on its own accord. 'Peel off a two inch slice of apple, bend in half with the skin sides together till the juice appears, then press on the eye lids gently. The redness goes and so does the pus – not completely but it is kept in check if done several times a day.' Yvonne Wilson from London.

Urine: Urine may seem an unlikely home remedy for conjunctivitis, but urine eyedrops are a particularly appropriate way of making use of its anti-infective properties. 'Applying a few drops of fresh or boiled urine can be very helpful in cases of conjunctivitis. It is sometimes wise to dilute the urine used for eyedrops with a bit of water.' Coen van der Kroon, *The Complete Guide to Urine Therapy*.

ALLERGIC CONJUNCTIVITIS

The best treatment is undoubtedly the anti-allergic compounds Opticrom or Predsol, but warm water compresses as described for infective conjunctivitis can help relieve the symptoms of grittiness and itchiness.

IRRITATIVE CONJUNCTIVITIS

Inadvertently rubbing the eye after having handled a chilli can cause intense pain and copious tears. Dr Richard Roberts, a genetic specialist in Texas and self-confessed chilli addict, describes the following interesting remedy: 'I once experienced the symptoms when in the company of several Mexican friends who urged me to put hair in the affected eye immediately. Though incredulous I grabbed for my wife's hair – his own was too short for the purpose – and the pain and tears cleared immediately. I cannot explain this effect.'

Constipation

Constipation is among the commonest and curiously the most debilitating of simple ailments,

Constipation

and often associated with a general sense of lethargy and melancholy. The pursuit of regularity therefore, besides relieving abdominal discomfort and colicky pains, has a noticeably euphoric effect. The reason is not clear. There is no doubt that a good 'bowel action' is satisfactory primarily due to the sense of evacuation but also because the anus is richly supplied with nerve fibres which are stimulated when the bowel opens, resulting in a most pleasing sensation. Further, the internal cleansing of the bowel with enemas or colonic irrigation is reputedly very pleasurable. The British journalist, Ysenda Maxton-Graham described it as 'the most satisfying loo going experience of my life. Years of stored up wind and matter such as old pips, stones and undigested pills are dispensed with – it is a joy to say goodbye to them.'

The colon is in a state of constant movement as contractions of the muscles in the wall impel the contents forwards. During an attack of constipation the colon is relatively inert and 'stimulant laxatives' are the traditional remedies. Mr Allan Wilson from Perthshire who practised as a pharmacist in Selkirk in the 1930s recalls:

'I am seventy-eight. As a teenager my mother would place two or three senna pods in half a cup of water, leaving to soak overnight and then drinking the water in the morning, convinced this "infusion" kept her regular. About the same time, my grandfather, then in his eighties, described taking a dose of extract of cascara sagrada liquid. It seemed to work for him. My aunt, with whom I resided at the time, also thought it good for me but I found it absolutely horrid to take, with an aftertaste that lasted for hours.'

These stimulant laxatives, such as senna and Epsom salts, have fallen out of fashion in recent years and prolonged use is now recognised to cause

48

the bowels to become dependent and indeed may
lead to permanent damage.

The alternative approach, and this really only
applies to those who are chronically constipated, is
to improve the regularity of the bowel by 'exercis-
ing' it. The presence of faecal matter in the colon
encourages colonic contractions, so the more faecal
matter that is present, the greater the amount of
exercise and thus the stronger, and 'fitter', the
bowel becomes.

As the two major constituents of faecal matter
are water and indigestible cellulose or 'fibre', then
the simplest of home remedies is to increase the
amount consumed.

WATER

The water content of the stool is reabsorbed as it
passes down the colon, thus the higher the water
intake, the less that needs to be reabsorbed and the
larger the bulk of the stool. Mrs Barbara Willett
from Cornwall reports: 'I became very constipated
when pregnant with my first child in 1956. My
family doctor advised "on waking in the morning
drink half to a pint of warm water and then lie on
your right side for about twenty minutes". This has
worked for me all my life – I do not necessarily
remain on my right side but I always drink the
water. I am seventy-five now and continue to find
it infallible. Many of my friends have benefited
from this advice.'

The temperature of the water, another corre-
spondent pointed out, is important as 'neither cold
nor hot water works. It has to be luke warm'. Mrs
Louise Dawson from Gloucestershire suggests a
variant of this remedy; 'cabbage water in which a
cabbage has been boiled for ten to fifteen minutes'.
It is, she says, 'quite pleasant with just salt and
pepper – but if desired add a little Marmite or

Bovril.' The alternative to warm water first thing in the morning is to drink less tea and coffee. Both are natural diuretics increasing the quantity of urine that is passed which is dehydrating. This increases the amount of water that needs to be reabsorbed from the stool which in turn decreases its bulk. Ms P. Austin from Middlesex writes: 'I cut down on tea and coffee gradually and increased my intake of plain water until the problem went away. Now, so long as I drink more plain water than tea and coffee every day I am not constipated.'

FIBRE

There is no doubt that increasing the bulk of the stool promotes its passage down the colon. This was convincingly shown in experiments conducted by Dr Denis Burkitt who compared the speed with which marker pellets were eliminated in a group of English school boys on a typical school diet with a similar number of Africans consuming plants and cereals all rich in 'dietary fibre'. The average African stool weighs between 300–500 grammes and takes 36 hours to pass, compared to that of the school boys which weighed between 100–150 grammes and took twice as long to pass down the colon.

There is nothing intrinsically desirable in passing a large stool especially if it requires consuming a rather dismal 'African-style' diet. Nonetheless, as is now well known, many (if not all) of those with constipation do benefit from increasing the amount of fibre in their diet by increasing the quantity of fruit and vegetables consumed, and by eating bran-based cereals and wholemeal bread. It is important to recognise, however, that this 'high fibre' diet is not suitable for everyone and can cause flatulence, abdominal distension and colicky pains.

NATURAL LAXATIVES

Prunes: The laxative property of prunes has been recognised for a long time and were described by the first radio doctor, Charles Hill, as 'nature's little workers'. Following intensive research conducted by Dr Sidney Masri of the United States Department of Agriculture, the active ingredient was identified as the chemical magnesium. In her book *The Food Pharmacy* Jean Carper notes 'when researchers removed the magnesium phosphate from prunes, the fruit's laxative properties dropped to zero but when they fed the powerful prune magnesium alone to mice not much happened either. It seems the famous prune chemical works only when it is in the prunes'. Those unaccustomed to eating prunes may initially experience symptoms similar to those experienced with a high fibre diet – flatulence and abdominal distension – but the intestinal tract usually adapts within a few weeks.

Sugar: Sugar attracts water and thus generates a loose stool. Babies with constipation respond well to bottled water to which a spoonful of brown sugar has been added. In adults honey has been shown to have a similar effect.

Beer: Beer drinkers do not suffer from constipation probably because beer combines both a high fluid intake and laxative properties of the sugars of fermented alcohol.

Some people find that one particular food, though not generally recognised as having laxative properties, nonetheless works for them. These include:

Cashew Nuts: 'I have been constipated all my life but at a rather boring cocktail party I sat near a small table on which was a saucer of cashew nuts. With nothing better to do I absent-mindedly nibbled a few. Next morning I had a beautiful easy motion – such a luxurious surprise that I tried to pin down the cause of it and decided it could only be the cashew nuts. I now take a small handful (ten to twelve) every day just before lunch. I have never looked back, and I adore cashew nuts anyway.' Mrs Irene Evans from West Glamorgan.

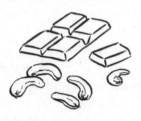

Chocolate: 'My mother, who lived to be ninety-nine, never travelled without a supply of Cadbury's Bourneville chocolate – her cure for constipation.' Mrs David Hilton from Kent.

Aloe vera: 'After suffering from constipation for nearly forty years I have tried enormous quantities of fruit, vegetables, water and fibre to no avail. I then read about aloe vera – the nineties wonder cure. Half a small liqueur glass either on rising or last thing at night works wonders. It bulks out the stool and gives an easy motion twice a day.' Anon.

In addition Mrs P. Whetton from Lincoln recommends five to six slices of beetroot twice a week and Mrs Kathleen Macdonald finds extra strong peppermint capsules – one or two a day – before meals 'excellent for constipation'.

Massage: Mr Michael Keef from Herefordshire writes: 'Find a good physiotherapist and get him or her to give a course of stomach massage. My late wife was cured from chronic constipation over a period of six months with a massage once a fortnight. This is better than all the other remedies.'

Coughs

Standard cough remedies are of two sorts – expectorants which seek to loosen the secretions in the lungs so they can be coughed up – or suppressants – which attempt to suppress the cough as their name suggests. There are several household remedies which can also be categorised in the same way, and included amongst the most unusual to feature in this anthology are noxious fumes from gas works or road building. There is considerable overlap here with the cold remedies and readers are referred to that section where appropriate.

Steam: Steam is a useful expectorant as well as soothing to irritated airways (see Colds).

Chicken soup: Chicken soup increases the velocity of nasal and bronchial secretions and thus is a particularly effective remedy for a dry cough (see Colds).

Noxious fumes: Noxious fumes were used as a common treatment for the persistent cough of whooping cough in childhood. Particularly favoured were the smells from gasworks, the smoke from a steam engine and liquid tar. 'When I was a little girl at infant school about seventy years ago and contracted whooping cough it was thought desirable for a child to inhale the sulphurous fumes coming from the local gasworks. I was taken daily for a walk past Chelmsford gasworks and instructed to inhale deeply. It certainly did the trick.' Miss I. E. Woolford from Chelmsford.

The gasworks remedy did not work for Mrs Elizabeth Jones from Dorset so her father resorted to more drastic measures: 'This necessitated a train journey through the Severn Tunnel. As soon as the train entered the tunnel my father opened the window and thrust my head out facing the engine. I have often thought that had a train been passing in the opposite direction, my cough might have been silenced permanently.'

The fumes from liquid tar would have worked in a similar way as this anonymous contributor points out: 'When I was young in the thirties in a North London suburb the recognised palliative for a cough was to locate an area where street resurfacing was taking place. I have clear memories of being daily walked up and down past the roadside brazier where a cauldron of tar was being prepared and required to deeply inhale the coal tar fumes.'

Cough medicine: Mr Norman Gardiner from Chelsea records this home-made cough syrup from the 'hungry Thirties': 'Sliced swede with brown sugar and placed between two plates in a warm place near the kitchen range. The juice exuded was used as a cough syrup.' In a variant of this recipe onion is substituted for the swede.

Wet towels: A nocturnal cough in a child, especially if he also coughs following exercise, is usually a sign of mild asthma which usually responds to appropriate anti-asthma medication. There may, however, be a simpler explanation and Mrs Bolt from Yorkshire suggests that central heating may, by drying the air, cause chronic nocturnal coughs in children. 'A wet towel over the radiator or a bowl of water brings immediate relief,' she writes.

A handkerchief: Cold air can irritate the airways resulting in a chronic cough at night for those who sleep in cold bedrooms. Mrs J. Barton from Sussex reports discovering the following remedy: 'As I coughed only at night for two winters, I thought if I could breathe warm air at night it would help. I put my head under the bedclothes and the coughing stopped – but began again when I came up for air. The next night I put a large thin handkerchief over my whole face and breathed in and out deeply through the mouth. I think the warm air breathed out slightly warmed the cold air going in.'

Cuts

There is only one immediate remedy for a bleeding cut and that is to apply pressure either by placing a clean handkerchief or tissue over the cut or, if it is long, by pushing the sides together between the thumbs of both hands. Cobwebs are reputed to stop bleeding but this is a diversion and anyhow they are difficult to find in sufficient quantities to be of any use. If, after half an hour, the bleeding persists, a tight bandage should be applied and medical attention should be sought urgently. Once the bleeding has stopped the question arises whether the cut is sufficiently wide to warrant stitching and if there is any doubt then again a visit to the casualty department is called for. For small cuts, however, various remedies can promote rapid healing.

Soap and water: The cut should be washed and any sand or grit removed. This reduces the risk of infection and prevents the discoloration or tattooing effect when small foreign bodies are left behind.

Egg membrane: Mrs Helen Cooper from Wareham describes this interesting alternative to the modern steri-strip: 'When I was ten years old I cut my eye just below the brow on the outer side. My mother cracked open an egg, removed a piece of the white membrane from the inside of the shell, and after cleaning the wound, placed the membrane over the cut. As it dried, so it pulled the cut together and eventually the membrane became quite hard when it was removed revealing a healed wound underneath.'

Honey: Honey has potent healing properties. Mrs M. S. Geering from Hertfordshire reports: 'Cuts, especially those caused when a knife slips, are easily and quickly cured by covering them with a coat of honey, pushing the edges together and covering it with an Elastoplast. A small cut will in this way heal overnight.'

Saliva: Saliva's curative potential is particularly appropriate for cuts and wounds. Mrs Pamela Betts from Leicestershire believes the phrase 'kissing better' probably comes from the instinct to lick wounds. 'Ever since my daughter was a baby, I have licked any minor cuts and abrasions she has incurred. As long as this was done within twenty minutes, the wound healed quickly without any infection.'

Dogs lick their cuts and wounds and it is possible that the healing properties of canine saliva might be even more marked than that of humans. As Mrs Gill McAnnee of Herefordshire discovered after she trod on an upturned tumbler which caused a deep cut to her foot. 'I am the sort of person who will never go to the doctor' she says, and so she hobbled around in pain for several weeks. Then one evening as she was watching television one of her dogs started licking the wound. By the following morning a scab had formed – and by the end of the week the cut had healed.

Cystitis

Cystitis is among the commonest of infections and all women probably know the following simple remedies which are included here. Increasing the fluid intake to 'flush out' the bladder and reducing the acidity of the urine with one or other of the alkaline type compounds available from the chemist are useful. Persistent or severe attacks require antibiotics which will also prevent the infection spreading up to the kidneys.

Water: Drinking two or three litres of water over twenty-four hours will increase the urine flow. It is advised that enough should be drunk to make the urine a pale yellow colour. In addition, a hot bath is very effective in relieving the pain of cystitis.

Alkalis: The burning sensation of cystitis is due to the acidity of the urine and is neutralised by one and a half teaspoonfuls of bicarbonate of soda in water or, if preferred, soda water or one or other of the proprietary preparations available from the chemist.

Cranberry juice: There is good evidence that cranberry juice prevents bacteria sticking to the wall of the bladder. Ocean Spray is a good brand of pure juice, unmixed with anything else. Dr A. E. Sobota from Ohio comments:

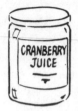

'The potential use of cranberry juice in the treatment of urinary tract infections might be particularly beneficial in the management of those who suffer recurrent infections. Long term preventative measures with antibiotics present several problems including toxicity, side effects and the emergence of resistant bacteria. In contrast cranberry juice is well accepted and no clinical side effects have been observed.'

For those particularly prone to recurrent infections the following two suggestions may prove useful.

Sex: Sexual intercourse encourages the passage of bacteria up the urethra to cause bladder infections, so it is probably advisable to pass urine soon after intercourse – and for the fastidious – before as well.

Diaphragms and tampons: The insertion of diaphragms and tampons into the vagina may increase the risk of cystitis. It is worth considering alternative forms of contraception and a sanitary towel should be used instead of tampons.

Deafness

Oscar Wilde's father, Sir William Wilde, was a distinguished ear surgeon in Dublin. He once observed in an epigram his son would have been proud of, 'there are only two types of deafness – one is due to earwax and is curable. The other is not due to wax and is not curable.' This is no longer strictly true as deafness in children in particular may be due to glue ear and cured by the insertion of grommets. Nonetheless, earwax overwhelmingly remains the commonest cause for deafness and certainly the most easily treatable.

Earwax is a remarkable substance with anti-infective properties which prevent bacterial and other infections taking hold in what would other-wise be a particularly suitable environment for infection, as the earhole is both dark and moist. Probably the most important home remedy is the injunction to resist the temptation to twizzle cot-ton buds into the ears as this only pushes the earwax further down and makes it more difficult to retrieve.

The solution for deafness due to earwax is to remove it, using the following procedure;

Olive oil: Olive oil moistens and loosens up the earwax and should be instilled in the ear for five consecutive days before attempting syringing the ear with water.

Water and syringe: There are few things quite as satisfying for a doctor than syringing out a pair of ears blocked by wax. In goes the stream of water. Out comes a brown oily glob, the deafness is miraculously cured and the pristine earhole looks clean enough to dine off. It is not a good idea to try this on oneself but a Canadian physician, Dr Maurice Ernis, describes how he treated himself while he was on holiday. While learning to windsurf some water shifted the wax in his ear so it became 'quite uncomfortable or worrisome, with hearing loss'. He goes on to say:

'This sort of thing spoils one's day and a lot of time is spent opening one's mouth as wide as one can in order to equalise the air pressure on both sides of the drum. On a trip to a local grocery store I saw a yellow refillable ketchup bottle of the plastic squeeze type and this seemed like a possible instrument for the job at hand. With one hand I squeezed the bottle full of warm water about two or three times, several pieces of wax were removed and my hearing returned to normal.'

Dry Mouth

A dry mouth due to paucity of saliva may be part of a generalised illness or a feature of 'old age'. It is a most distressing condition making eating difficult and causing chronic dental problems as saliva is essential to oral hygiene. There are luckily several synthetic saliva preparations available form the chemist and a former pharmacist, Mr S. Greening-Jackson from Nottinghamshire, recommends potassium iodide dispensed as mist.pod.iod.ammon.bnf. Mr Paul Goriup from East Sussex makes the following observation – firstly that red wine drunk in the evening can cause dry mouth at night and secondly that central heating can have a similar effect by drying up the air for which the antidote is to place a bowl of water in each room.

Two contributors submitted unusual remedies which they maintain stimulate saliva production.

String: When Mrs Gogi Younger from Manchester discovered this treatment, her doctor advised that she should patent it: 'I put a bit of thread in my mouth, usually a small bit of thickish cotton scrunched up into a small ball and leave in my mouth and cheek usually changing a few times a day. I carry my cut off bits of string in my handbag at home and am never without. I have accidentally swallowed the occasional small bit of thread many times and it has done no harm. This remedy has certainly changed my life.'

Paper hanky: Mr M. Nichols from Kent describes his remedy as follows: 'Cut a strip off a paper handkerchief one and a quarter inches by approximately five inches and roll it up. Place it along the front of the mouth between the teeth. Close the mouth. Gently press the paper between the teeth while using the tip of the tongue to rotate the paper. After repeating these movements several times, the paper does seem to activate the moisture in the mouth.'

Eye Grit

The tissues in front of the eye – the cornea – are the most sensitive anywhere in the body for the obvious reason that were they to be damaged by a foreign body, it might seriously impair one's vision. The pain caused by eye grit is thus of such intensity that it requires the immediate removal of the offending object. There are a variety of methods of achieving this.

The tongue: Mr S. J. Green from Swansea recalls: 'My mother took my head in her hands, telling me to hold my head back. She then pulled up my eyelids and with her tongue licked over the ball of my eye, removing the offending piece of grit.'

Castor oil: Mrs Cynthia Castellan from Staffordshire comments: 'When the children had a sand-pit, I always kept castor oil handy for floating out sand in the eyes – also a bottle of witchhazel to soothe them afterwards (diluted on damp cottonwool).'

Hair: This remedy comes from Mr Bill Annable from Nottinghamshire:

> 'Stand in front of the patient, remove from your head a long, strong hair. If you have not one borrow one from your patient or someone else close by as the hair must be strong. Make a loop with the hair. Hold the loop between the thumb and forefinger of the hand you are to use. The loop should ideally be three-eighths of an inch or less sticking out from the thumb and forefinger. With the thumb of the other hand lift or lower the eyelid in question. Ask the patient to look in the direction that exposes the debris. Let the loop or hair manoeuvre or scoop the debris away. When you have done this a few times, the debris is out in seconds. The hair does not irritate the eye and the patient has no feeling that something is being poked into the eye.'

Eye Strain

Eye strain is commonly due to reading in poor light or to uncorrected short sightedness. In this case the solution is quite straightforward – read in a good light, visit the optician to have your eyes tested and buy a decent pair of glasses. The symptoms of eye strain have become more common in recent years due to the introduction of the VDU. Here the following remedies may be of help.

Close the eyes: There are many times during the working day, speaking on the telephone for example, when it is not necessary to watch the VDU screen. This provides an opportunity to rest the eyes whilst simultaneously bathing them in a soothing tear secretion. This can be done by simply closing the eyes. Depending on how much time is spent on the phone this simple suggestion can rest the eyes for one or two hours a day.

Tea: Tea is reported to be an excellent antidote for eye strain. Mrs Patricia O'Driscoll from London describes the method she favours: 'My remedy is cold or tepid tea from the bottom of a teapot, so it is really "stewed". Straining it into a bowl will filter out the tea leaves. Then bathe the eyes with it. Alternatively soak a pad and leave it over the eyes for half an hour or so securing it in place with a few twists of a crepe bandage. Freshly brewed tea is not as effective, so leave it in the pot between cups of tea and it gathers strength.' No doubt tepid teabags directly applied to the eye might have a similar effect.

Massage: It is inadvisable to rub sore tired eyes as they will then become swollen and red and drag the surrounding skin. Two types of simple massage can, however, be very restful as described by Jill Nice in her book *Herbal Remedies*. The first is palming: 'Press the base of the palms of the hands gently but firmly over the closed eyes and maintain pressure for several minutes.' The second is finger massage: 'Using a little fine oil and the tops of three fingers stroke gently from the bridge of the nose out across the eyes beneath and above the brows several times.

With finger and thumb pinch the nose beneath the bridge and maintain the pressure for several seconds.'

Foreign Bodies

The two orifices into which small children have a tendency to stuff foreign bodies – beads, sponge, crumbs, sweets and much else besides – are the nose and the ear. These can be difficult to remove, necessitating long hours waiting in casualty, and so it is worth trying one or two of the following manoeuvres.

The nose: The presence of a foreign body up the nose can give rise to the most unpleasant of fetid body odours. Dr Michael Farnham, a paediatrician in Miami, describes a typical case: 'For a couple of months a two-year-old child had suffered from a body odour so unpleasant that the teacher at her nursery school insisted she be removed – even the child's mother could not stand to be near her. A thorough examination of the nose disclosed a piece of bathroom sponge with the same foul odour as that coming from the child. In an hour of its removal, the body odour had disappeared.'

Dr Eugene Guazzo, an American paediatrician has perfected a technique for removing unwanted objects from nostrils. His method is as follows: 'Place one's mouth over that of the child and blow gently until a degree of resistance is felt, then give one sharp exhalation, the object should pop out.' This should be carried out under medical supervision as it may be unsuitable in some cases.

The ear: Foreign objects buried deep in the ear present more of a challenge. Dr Mason Thompson from Georgia describes the following procedure which may be attempted if the object can be seen under a good light:

> 'I have removed small, hard objects, particularly the elusive sliding plastic bead, from the canal by using glue applied to a straightened paper clip. The procedure is accomplished by merely wetting the end of the paper clip with a small amount of rapidly drying glue; the object is visualised and the moistened tip of the paper clip is then placed against it. One waits a few seconds for drying and slowly withdraws the foreign body from the canal. The sliding hard object is more easily removed by this procedure whereas the embedded object may not be.'

Again, this should be attempted only under medical supervision.

The ear may also provide a comfortable home for small creatures that crawl into it at night and prove difficult to dislodge. This certainly does require a visit to the casualty department though the question of the best method of removal is offered here as one of the more diverting medical experiments of recent times. Numerous methods have been described for removing the common cockroach from the ear canal, the most popular of which appears to be placing mineral oil in the canal and the subsequent manual removal of the creature. More recently, the local anaesthetic lignocaine spray has been suggested as a more effective approach to the problem.

> 'Recently a patient presented with a cockroach in both ears and it was recognised immediately that fate had granted us the opportunity for an elegant comparative trial. We placed the time tested mineral oil in one ear canal and the cockroach succumbed after a valiant but futile struggle and its

removal required much dexterity. In the opposite ear we sprayed 2 per cent lignocaine solution. The response was immediate; the cockroach exited the canal at a convulsive speed and attempted to escape across the floor. A fleetfooted doctor promptly applied an equally time-tested remedy and killed the creature using the simple crush method.'

Dr K. O'Toole from the university of Pittsburgh suggests this small experiment 'provides further evidence to justify the use of lignocaine for the treatment of the problem that has bugged mankind throughout recorded history'.

Hair Problems

When a child's hair or eyelashes become plastered together with chewing gum or plasticine, the instinctive reaction is to wash it with shampoo – but to no avail. There might seem no alternative other than to cut away the matted hair. But there is chocolate.

From personal experience Dr J. H. Marks, a physician in South Africa, noticed that chewing gum dissolved in the mouth if chocolate is eaten at the same time: 'Following this lead I have repeatedly removed chewing gum from hair by rubbing in soft melted chocolate and allowing it to dry. After this the hair is washed well and the chocolate and the gum come away together.'

Several other gum removing remedies have also been recommended including peanut butter and hair lacquer. 'The propellant "freezes" the gum and after a couple of minutes it can be taken out of the hair quite easily' reports Mr Stephen Jessop from West Sussex. (This of course should not be used on eyelashes.)

For dry hair there are shelves full of conditioners available from the local chemist, but two home remedies are sometimes used. The first is mayonnaise which can be left on the hair for up to an hour before washing out and the second is beer sprayed onto the hair after it has been shampooed and dried.

Heartburn

Heartburn is a most distressing problem. It is caused by weakness of the band of muscle that separates the stomach from the oesophagus (whose purpose is to prevent acidic secretions regurgitating back upwards). While standing, there may no problem, but as soon as the head hits the pillow at night the corrosive acidic juices – capable of dissolving a lump of meat in a couple of hours – surge upwards into the oesophagus causing enough discomfort to render sleep impossible.

For many, heartburn drags on for years, waxing and waning for no apparent reason. Luckily, there is now a range of treatments available from the chemist which either singly, or in combination, make this one of the more treatable of chronic gut problems. These include antacids that neutralise the acidic secretions, and drugs such as Gaviscon that create a raft of viscous material floating on top of the stomach contents. Alternatively, it is possible to 'turn off' the acidic secretions with drugs such as Tagamet – better known for the treatment of ulcers. A third approach is to accelerate the emptying of the stomach contents so that there is less acid to reflux upwards using drugs like Maxolon – though this requires a doctor's prescription.

Heartburn may also be alleviated by several types of home remedy.

Bricks: Bricks placed under the head of the bedstead to a height of twenty centimetres can, by preventing the upward flow of the gastric juices, markedly reduce the severity of heartburn. Dr M. F. Paterson from Hertfordshire reports that her husband found this much more efficacious than standard medical treatment and 'he was immediately free from nocturnal pains'.

Loose trousers: Dr Octavia Bessa of Stamford, Connecticut, has identified tight trousers as a cause of abdominal discomfort and heartburn. 'Tight trouser syndrome' he reports, 'is a self-induced medical problem which interferes with the forward propulsion of the stomach contents.' The cure is a larger pair of trousers, supported if necessary by a pair of braces.

Cream: Cream has antacidic properties. 'After suffering from debilitating heartburn for many

years I found that cream taken at breakfast, a tablespoonful in each of two cups of coffee, completely obviates the need to take antacids. The cream taken at breakfast is effective for 24 hours', writes Mr A. C. H. Brent-Good from the Isle of Wight.

Alcohol: It is advisable to reduce alcohol intake, especially in the evening, as this relaxes the muscle between the stomach and oesophagus resulting in heartburn. An interesting and unexplained exception is cider, or cider vinegar, which appears to have a protective effect. Mrs S. Cortis from Devon reports that her husband's heartburn has been successfully treated with cider. 'He drinks a tumbler each evening with his meal and since doing so has had no problem with acidic secretion. He finds the non-fizzy type best.'

Hiccoughs

There were, at the last count, over a hundred 'cures' for hiccoughs, ranging from sipping water to massaging the rectum. Meanwhile, the well-publicised case of a man who had been hiccoughing for six years generated 60,000 letters of advice. This profusion of remedies reflect the fact that there is no sure-fire remedy for intractable hiccoughs, though conversely, mild attacks can be terminated by many different manoeuvres. The source of hiccoughs is the contraction of the muscles of the diaphragm – the sheet of muscle between the lungs and the chest – which expel air from the lungs which is then abruptly blocked by closure of the vocal chords.

There are three main groups of remedies, all of which seek to eliminate the muscular contractions of the diaphragm. The first is to physically suppress the movement of the diaphragm. The second involves stimulating the uvula – the fleshy protuberance at the back of the throat which, according to Dr Janet Travel, the world expert on hiccoughs and formerly physician to President Kennedy, is a main trigger point for hiccoughs. The third is to counteract the action of the nerves that supply the diaphragm and cause muscular contractions. The following list of remedies falls broadly into these three categories.

Hiccoughs

Breath holding: Everyone knows this remedy – hold your breath and count to forty. The reason why breath holding works is not clear, though it may be that by increasing the carbon dioxide in the blood it reduces the irritability of the diaphragm muscle. The same effect can be achieved more readily by rebreathing into a paper bag.

Splint the diaphragm: Pull the knees up into the chest or just lean forwards.

Sip water: There are three variants of this. 'My mother used to make me stand, bend over a glass of water and take a few sips from the wrong (far) side of the glass. My husband is a retired GP and can't understand why it works – but it does.' Mrs Jill Mendel from Middlesex.

'Hold nose, press ear flaps to close ear canal, and drink from a cup of water – thus holding one's breath (some assistance may be required).' Anon.

'Take a sip of water and say a word (any word) out loud. Repeat several times until the hiccoughs stop. We were taught this as children and our word was "tiger". We had a cat of that name, or maybe it was "Tiger Tim's Weekly", a favourite children's comic.' Miss A. Powell from Herefordshire.

Stimulate the uvula: There are several suggested way of doing this, including pulling forcibly on the tongue, stroking the back of the throat with a spoon or cottonbud, or swallowing dry granulated sugar or a lemon wedge soaked in angostura bitters.

Nerve stimulation: The nervous system that controls the diaphragm can be stimulated by compressing the eyeballs or massaging the neck – or using the most unusual of hiccoughs remedies – massaging the rectum. Dr Francis Fesmire of the

University Hospital in Cap Florida explains:

> 'A 27-year-old man came to the emergency
> department with intractable hiccoughs for 72
> hours. Initially gagging and tongue pulling
> manoeuvres were attempted, followed by eye-
> ball compression and massaging of the side of the
> neck (the carotid sinus). Rectal massage with a
> finger was then attempted using a slow circum-
> ferential motion. The frequency of the hiccoughs
> immediately began to slow and terminated within
> 30 seconds.'

Infant Colic

Human babies cry far longer and more loudly than
the offspring of any other species, and sound levels
have been recorded of 117 decibels which is only
just less than that of a pneumatic drill. Compared
with the other abilities of small infants, this vocal
facility is exceptionally highly developed both in
power and duration, and no doubt for good reasons.
It is not enough for the baby to alert its parents to
the need to be fed or changed, their lives have to be
made sufficiently unpleasant to force them to react
– and very effective it is too.

Regrettably, some infants cannot be consoled.
This is the nightmare of young parents whose
difficult babies cry inconsolably for hours at a time,
particularly in the evenings and despite every
conceivable attention. Typically the baby draws up
its legs, clenches its fists and emits high pitched
screams for several minutes, stops for a while and
then starts again. This is infant colic and the
question of its cause has, over the years, generated
an enormous number of fanciful theories: the
babies are overfed or underfed, or fed the wrong

things; they suffer from an allergy, or heightened muscle tones; the fault lies with the parents who 'pick the baby up too much', or 'bounce it too much after its feed'. It has even been suggested that persistent crying by the baby is a form of malingering.

The popularity of such explanations is all the more remarkable because over a decade ago Professor R. S. Illingworth from Sheffield University convincingly showed that the reason for this persistent crying in infancy was that the baby was in pain induced by intestinal spasms. Everything fits this explanation: the rhythmical paroxysms of screaming, the accompanying loud bowel sounds and the temporary cessations following the passage of wind. Convincingly Professor Illingworth showed that the anti-spasmodic drug dicyclomine was 'strikingly successful' in preventing these attacks. Regrettably this drug is no longer available to be prescribed to young babies following some poorly substantiated reports of adverse reactions, so parents must now soldier on with less effective remedies. The following have been recommended:

Spin dryer: Placing the colicky crying baby in its carrycot on the spin dryer is well recognised to have a soothing effect. The reason is not clear but the baby is presumably relaxed by the rhythmic movement of the dryer.

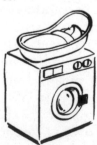

A spin in a car: For similar reasons as with the spin dryer, parents find that taking the baby for a drive during a colicky attack can be remarkably effective.

Alcohol: A small dose of alcohol has been recommended which presumably relaxes the smooth muscle of the gut, preventing the build up of wind that contributes to the colicky attack.

Infertility

As virtually all couples trying to have a child will have conceived within a year, it is likely that failure to do so within this time means that there is a fertility problem. The woman may not be ovulating, or there may be a physical impediment such as blocked fallopian tubes preventing the sperm reaching the egg. Alternatively the man may have a low sperm count. Sorting out what is precisely amiss – and how to put it right – is not necessarily very complex but requires specialist help, so there is not much that a couple can do on their own to increase the likelihood of successful conception. The following suggestions may, however, be useful.

The woman can buy a special kit from the chemist to ascertain that she is ovulating and if this is the case then it is appropriate to ensure that intercourse takes place most frequently around this time – in the middle of the menstrual cycle usually two weeks after the cessation of her monthly period.

The cause of infertility on the male side – a low sperm count – is readily determined by performing a semen analysis. There may be several reasons for this – one of which, the temperature in the scrotum, can be treated by a simple home remedy.

Cold water: A cool ambient temperature is necessary for adequate sperm production – which is why the testes are conveniently placed outside the body. Ideally, to increase sperm numbers it would be desirable to enhance this effect by keeping the testes artificially cool throughout the day. Urologists have been working on a device that might achieve this – a sort of glorified jock strap through which cold water circulates continuously. Regrettably the prototype seems to have an insuperable design defect which results in the steady drip of icy water down the wearer's leg. A simple alternative is to immerse the scrotum in a large cup of cold water three times a day for at least ten minutes. The result has been described by Mrs Ann Claxton from Bristol:

> 'My husband was told he was almost completely infertile by a fertility expert. His sperm count was 2.5 million per millilitre which was described as "grossly abnormal . . . fertility must be low if present at all". He was advised to spray his testicles for ten minutes morning and evening with cold water and to wear loose underpants. Within three months his sperm count had risen to 56 million, and I subsequently had three pregnancies in five years – two at the first attempt.'

Abstention: Frequent intercourse naturally depletes the absolute sperm count as it does not have time to recover. Theoretically therefore relative abstention should, by allowing the number of sperm to recover, boost the chances of successful conception. This has been confirmed by doctors of the university of California's Medical Center. Ten men were asked to produce sperm samples after periods of abstention allocated at random. Results were dramatic. An average sperm count of 60 million per millilitre soared to 130 million after a week's abstention and the total semen volume doubled to 4 millilitres. Thus it would appear that when it comes to conceiving there can be little doubt that the male can try too hard.

Insect Bites

There is a wide range of proprietary preparations available from the chemist both to prevent and treat insect bites. In addition Mrs E. Eardill from County Down recommends Bonjela: 'it forms a skin almost like clingfilm and stops the intense itching.'

Two home remedies have also been suggested.

Toothpaste: Mrs Linda Williams from St Albans reports that toothpaste topically applied stops the itching: 'I was told this in Botswana and have used it ever since.'

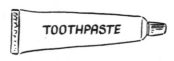

Hot water: Mrs Geraldine Hobson from Dorset was taught this remedy by her great grandmother. 'Hold a flannel by the end under a very hot tap. Wring out thoroughly and then press onto the bite. It will be almost too hot to bear but, of course, do not scald yourself. Repeat if necessary. The bite will itch even more furiously as the inflammation is 'drawn-out' by the heat – but after this the result is miraculous. It is more effective than any lotion or potion you can buy.'

Insomnia

It is possible to get by with very little sleep. Leonardo da Vinci, it is claimed, trained himself to take a nap for fifteen minutes every four hours, ninety minutes in total leaving the other 22.5 hours of the day to spend productively painting and inventing. However, most people do need their usual seven or eight hours and the lives of insomniacs who are unable to achieve this can be fairly wretched. The proprietary preparation Nytol can be obtained from chemists without prescription and there are two types of home remedy, lettuce and sleep hygiene.

Lettuce: Mr J. Jolly from Cheshire describes his experience of the hypnotic qualities of lettuce: 'I was a housemaster at an approved school. My charges, boys of fifteen to sixteen age group were in dormitories for about twenty boys. The morning after having had a rather difficult "lights out" time with boys complaining about being unable to sleep, I was overheard by an elderly cook who excused herself and interrupted the conversation stating that the traditional remedy was to give them a lettuce leaf to eat.

'On my next evening duty shift I raided the pantry for the biggest lettuce leaves I could find and dished them out as required to the slow sleepers. Hey presto! It worked. Since then I have often wondered whether test match cricketers lunches of large salads are responsible for so many early afternoon dismissals.'

Sleep hygiene: Dr Colin Espie, clinical psychologist at the University of Glasgow, provides the following advice. It starts with elementary 'sleep hygiene'.

Exercise – late afternoon or early evening is best. Avoid exercise near bedtime. Fit people have better quality sleep.

Diet – snacks before bedtime should be light and fluid intake limited.

Caffeine – coffee, tea and 'cola' contain this; intake should be moderated.

Alcohol – regular use as an hypnotic disrupts sleeping patterns. A hot milky drink is preferable.

Environment – bed and mattress should be comfortable, room temperature should be around 65 degrees Fahrenheit.

Next it is necessary to establish an optimal sleeping pattern.

(i)   Go to bed only when you are 'sleepy tired' and not by conventional habit.

(ii) Put the light out immediately you retire.

(iii) Do not read or watch television in bed.

(iv) If you are not asleep within twenty minutes get out of bed and sit and relax in another room until you are 'sleepy tired' again.

(v)   Do not nap during the day.

(vi) Do not take recovery sleep to compensate for a previous bad night.

(vii) Follow the programme rigidly for several weeks to establish an efficient and regular pattern.

Finally, he gives advice on overcoming the two main impediments to sleep.

Tension: Practice a relaxation routine when in bed. Concentrate on breathing, try to breathe deeply and slowly. Tense and relax major voluntary muscles groups in turn interspersed with breathing exercises. The groups comprise arms, neck and shoulders, face and eyes, stomach, back and legs.

Intrusive thoughts: Tell yourself that 'sleep will come when it is ready', that 'relaxing in bed is almost as good'. Try to keep your eyes open in a darkened room and as they naturally try to close tell yourself to 'resist that just for another few seconds'. This procedure 'tempts' sleep to take over. Try to ignore irrelevant ideas and thoughts. Visualise a pleasing scene or try repeating a neutral word such as 'the' every few seconds.

Irritable Bowel Syndrome

The large bowel is in a state of constant movement, as the muscles in its wall contract and relax impelling its contents onwards. This wave-like motion is absent in those with irritable bowel syndrome who as a result suffer alternately from either constipation – where the bowel is inert – or diarrhoea – where it is overactive, with colicky pains and an excess of wind. No single cause has been identified, though the severity of the symptoms can be exacerbated by certain foods, while stress is certainly a contributory factor.

As there is no single cause of IBS, everyone's case is different, and finding the best treatment is very much a matter of trial and error. There are many proprietary preparations from the chemist for one or other of the several symptoms – laxatives for constipation, anti-diarrhoeal drugs for diarrhoea, charcoal tablets for wind and peppermint based products for colic.

None of the following remedies will therefore apply to all, but serve to illustrate the scope of possible treatments. Two relevant symptoms, constipation and wind, are considered elsewhere in this anthology in more detail.

Diet: There are two important aspects to the question of diet in irritable bowel syndrome. The first concerns the general advice that patients should seek to exercise their bowel with a 'high fibre' diet – with lots of unrefined cereals, brown bread, pasta and so on, supplemented if necessary by special fibre supplements or high fibre cereals. This increases the bulk of the stool and encourages the smooth wave-like motion of the bowel, while at the same time preventing constipation.

A high fibre diet is certainly effective in some cases, but in others it may exacerbate symptoms, particularly increasing the quantities of wind in the bowel and associated colicky pains. Those made worse should clearly try to reduce rather than increase the amount of fibrous food in their diet.

The second aspect of diet is that certain foods will either exacerbate, or in some cases dramatically relieve the condition. Finding out which food affects the bowel can really only be determined by personal experience.

The most common exacerbating foods include, as already mentioned, 'high fibre' foods like bread and cereals; flatus inducing foods of which the most notorious are beans but also include cabbages, Brussels sprouts, broccoli, cauliflower and onions; dairy products where the person is intolerant to the lactose they contain; spicy foods particularly chillies; and acidic foods, oranges, grapefruits and vinegary salad dressings; finally, coffee, which can directly influence the nerves controlling the muscles in the walls of the bowel.

Constipation: See under **Constipation**. In brief, the most important are water (lots of it); fibre (where appropriate) and natural laxatives such as sugar (or honey), prunes and cashew nuts.

Diarrhoea: There are several dietary remedies for

diarrhoea to be found in any book of herbal medicine including rice, oats and potatoes but none are nearly as effective as the proprietary remedies obtained from the chemist which are clearly to be preferred.

Wind: See under **Wind**. The main points are to avoid where possible wind-inducing foods, and if gas is trapped in the gut causing distension to try the 'Mecca position' to aid its expulsion (see p. 112).

Pain: The colicky pains of IBS are the symptoms that cause most distress. As with the treatment of diarrhoea, there are several home remedies including massaging the abdomen and the topical application of heat with a hot water bottle. But, once again, the treatments from the chemist, both painkillers and antispasmodics, are much more effective and thus to be preferred.

Itching

Itching is something of a medical mystery. It has some relationship to pain whose nerve fibres it shares, but whereas pain is useful in forcing one to withdraw from a painful stimulus, the instinctive response to an itch is to scratch – but to what end? Then there is the curious way that scratching or rubbing an itchy area not only brings relief but pleasure, so there is an urge to carry on, even though it is absolutely certain that once the relief has worn off, the itching will return with a vengeance.

There are four main types of itching. The first is that associated with some recognisable skin complaint such as athlete's foot, eczema, scabies and ringworm, for which the treatment is obviously for that of the underlying condition. Secondly, a generalised itching may be a response to some food or drink or to a change in physical environment. There are reports of people itching after drinking a glass of red wine, going for a run, having a hot bath, or even wearing elasticated knickers. Thirdly, there may be a hidden medical cause for generalised itching. The commonest is undoubtedly a side effect of some medication the patient is taking but both an 'over' – and an 'under' – active thyroid can cause itchiness, as can anaemia due to insufficient iron, and also diabetes, all of which will be diagnosed by appropriate blood tests. Very occasionally itching may be the first symptom of Hodgkin's Disease, preceding its appearance by a year or more.

The final type of itching is 'itching of unknown cause' to which the following remedies apply. Especially common in the older age group, there are two particularly virulent forms involving the anus and the vulva, known respectively as pruritus ani and pruritus vulvae respectively.

The general principle in treating these conditions is that the skin should not be exposed to hidden chemicals, so perfumed soaps and deodorants should be avoided. The skin should be kept moist, so emollient oils can be added to the bath or applied afterwards and these are readily available from local chemists. Lastly, a mild steroid ointment is often helpful, and this too can be purchased over the counter without a prescription.

Water: It is commonly believed that over-frequent bathing can exacerbate generalised itchiness. This now seems to be debatable but it would seem wise to bathe only in lukewarm water rather than hot, which is more likely to dry the skin out.

Hairdryers: Dry rubbing with a towel after a bath can exacerbate itchiness, particularly of the anal and vulval regions. It is recommended that these sites should preferably be dried with a hairdryer.

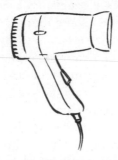

Urine: Urine contains the emollient urea and in the past builders and particularly bricklayers would wash their hands in urine to prevent the occupational dermatitis associated with handling bricks and mortar. Similarly mothers at one time would wipe their babies with their urine soaked nappies as it was believed to be good for the complexion. Adding a small amount of urine to the bath is a cheaper and more readily available alternative to the emollient oils purchased from the chemist.

Gloves: Gloves worn at night will prevent the excoriations of the skin caused by nocturnal scratching.

Clothes: Loose fitting cotton underwear should be worn next to the skin as man-made fibres can cause or exacerbate itchiness. A useful hint for women afflicted with pruritus vulvae is to cut the gusset out of their tights thus improving the circulation of air to the affected region.

Diet: Certain foods may exacerbate itchiness and their exclusion from the diet can bring blessed relief. It is well known that some cases of child eczema may respond dramatically to a dairy free diet. For reasons unknown, coffee is said to be an important exacerbating factor in pruritus ani and less convincingly beer, chocolate and tomato ketchup have been implicated in a similar way.

Migraine

There is no single cause of migraine. Many different factors can be involved in controlling the size of the arteries in the brain, whose initial constriction causes the warning symptoms, and whose subsequent dilation creates a crashing headache. It is not at all surprising that a treatment which works miraculously for one person might be ineffective for another. Standard medical drugs are certainly effective for many. Mrs Constance Benton from London reduced her monthly 96-hour ordeal to eight hours with Imigran injections. Mrs Marjorie Wells of Bristol reports that 'after years of migraine attacks and having every tablet' she found that Cafergot suppositories – combining caffeine and ergotamine – provided "instant relief".'

Three contributors discovered, by accident, that drugs taken for a different condition altogether combated their migraine. Mr Clive Mills from Nuneaton who has suffered migraines for 30 years says 'I used to lose three days of my life at ten day intervals'. Then he was given Diltiazem for his angina and has had no migraine attacks since. He writes that he can even 'eat chocolate and drink red wine with impunity'. Mr P. Mason found that Prozac had the same effect, and Mrs Penny Bullivant of Salisbury found that the betablockers she took for her raised blood pressure stopped her migraines immediately. In fact, betablockers are a well recognised migraine preventive treatment as indeed is a small dose of daily aspirin. Dr R. M. Miller of Sussex particularly recommends aspirin as being beneficial in a major attack, quite independent of its analgesic effects.

Two simple remedies suggest some relationship between stomach biliousness and migraine, where treating the former prevents the onset of the latter. Mr A. L. Baker of Dorset suggests a heaped teaspoon of Eno Fruit Salts in half a glass of water. Mrs Rosemary Stanbury of Swindon swears by the same thing in the form of two pints of soda water. She writes: 'within ten minutes the eyes are better and the following headache is negligible.'

Mrs Marianne Ticehurst from Essex observes: 'one of my many (symptoms) was a swollen left eye and congested left nostril.' She started to use the nasal decongestant Otrivine, right at the beginning of an attack – or when she anticipated one was on the way. She observed, 'gradually the attacks reduced in number and now I do not have migraines at all.'

Dentist, Mr Rory Linden-Kelly has discovered an association between migraine and increased muscle spasm around the jaw. The treatment involves wearing an acrylic appliance over the teeth at night to prevent the subconscious grinding habit. This reduces the muscle spasm and can prevent migraine.

Despite the disparate nature of these remedies a common theme seems to be that along with the well known dietary precipitants of migraine, disturbances in the stomach, nasal area and muscles may also be a contributory factor. Thus treatment directed at these areas may prove effective.

Night Cramps

Everyone gets night cramp from time to time which, if prolonged, propels the sufferer out of a warm bed to spend minutes walking up and down the bedroom floor. They become more frequent with the passage of years and, for those seriously afflicted, can disrupt a restful night's sleep. The pain is caused by acute spasm of the muscles and its cause is not known. Standard medical therapy is quinine sulphate tablets taken on retiring, though why it should work is not known.

There are a variety of home remedies including two of the most unusual in this collection – magnets and corks.

Tonic water: Tonic water contains quinine, and a tumblerful on retiring is reputed to be as effective as quinine sulphate tablets.

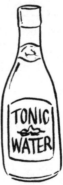

Pillows: Cramp sufferers are advised to keep their legs flexed by, for example, placing a pillow under the knee or against the foot. This prevents the leg muscles from relaxing completely and thus going into spasm.

Exercises: Lady Ford from East Lothian suggests

the following manoeuvre: 'Stand facing a wall about a yard away and place both arms flat against it. Brace legs, straighten knees and push hard ten times, then relax. Repeat two or three times.' Alternatively, Mr F. A. Murphy from Merseyside has a simpler suggestion: 'If you have cramp in the legs point the big toe upwards and it goes.'

Rebreathing: Miss R. T. Clark from Newmarket suggests a remedy similar to the 'paper bag cure' for hiccoughs. 'At the onset of leg cramp I cup my hands closely over mouth and nose and breathe deeply, thus reinhaling the exhaled breath. Gradually the inhaled carbon dioxide reaches the taut muscles and relaxes them. It may take forty to fifty breaths but it always works and the cramp does not return.'

Corks: Mrs M. S. Geering from Hertfordshire reports:

> 'Both my late husband and I used to have our sleep broken by cramps perhaps two or three times a week. When visiting my doctor on another matter I mentioned this to him and he suggested I put a cork under our mattress. This I did without telling my husband. Neither of us suffered cramp again. The first my husband knew about the cork was six months later when a dinner party guest mentioned he suffered from cramps and I passed this remedy on to him.'

This account is particularly compelling because it would appear the cork worked for Mrs Geering's husband even though he was unaware of its presence under the mattress. Mrs Angela Beckon from Huntingdon describes a similar instance where the remedy worked independently for both partners:

> 'Many years ago I was told to put a few corks beneath my mattress. It worked wonders. No more creeping out on the cold kitchen floor to alleviate it.

My husband did not believe in it until his leg cramp became more frequent – when he tried it too. Complete success. The ladies from the Social Services, however, did wonder whether the corks might have had something to do with secret drinking.'

If the cork is displaced for any reason, the remedy no longer appears to work. Mr Geoffrey Bellis from Wrexham describes how his wife was advised by a friend to place a cork in her bed – with excellent results. 'After a few months a severe attack of cramp caused her to doubt the efficacy of the advice she had been given. Surprise, surprise, when she later made the bed she found the two corks on the bedroom floor.'

Magnets: Mrs Hilary Bonye from Kent has found that magnets have worked to prevent her cramps for over twenty years.

'I put a magnet on the affected part of my leg and the pain disappears in a few seconds. My husband, a physicist, was doubtful at first, but he agrees the effectiveness of the treatment is no coincidence.'

Further, as with Mrs Bellis's experience, if the magnet is displaced, the remedy no longer works. Mrs Eileen Lynch from Suffolk uses a four inch magnet purchased from a toy shop:

'When I had a cramp again a few nights ago, I discovered the magnet had slipped down the side of the mattress.'

Nose Bleeds

To stop a nose bleed – as everyone knows – it is necessary to apply pressure, though the technique is important. The nose should be pinched forcefully between finger and thumb and held in that position for at least ten to fifteen minutes. For those prone to recurrent nose bleeds, the blood vessels on the inner surface of the nose need to be cauterised. While waiting for this procedure to be done, it may be sensible to purchase a swimmer's nose clip. Dr Philip Turner explains: 'This can be left in place for as long as necessary without causing too much discomfort. It does not cause the finger aching so common with manual compression. It is equally effective in children and adults and well tolerated by the younger patient.'

Piles

Piles, or haemorrhoids, are an affliction unique to humans and the roll call of famous sufferers include Martin Luther, Cardinal Richlieu, Copernicus and Casanova. Napoleon was a life-long sufferer and a particularly bad attack on the eve of Waterloo, it is alleged, was an important contributory factor to the defeat of his army by Wellington.

Piles are caused by the prolapse of the veins around the anal canal which are then pinched tight by the muscles of the anal sphincter, resulting in bleeding and intense pain. A standard treatment available from the chemist without prescription is a cream containing a mild steroid and a local anaesthetic such as Anugesic. There are in addition a range of home remedies that can be tried.

A hot bath: Hot baths can often cure a milder case of haemorrhoids and prevent their recurrence.

Ice: Cold constricts the blood vessels as well as having a local anaesthetic effect. The pile sufferer is advised to sit naked on a chair on which has been placed ice cubes (or a packet of frozen vegetables) wrapped in a clean towel.

Laxatives: Constipation can, by causing straining at stool, precipitate an attack of piles, while the pain of piles, by discouraging defecation, can cause constipation. In either situation, loosening the stool and increasing its bulk with a high intake of fluid and fibre is an appropriate treatment (see Constipation).

Vaseline: A thin layer of Vaseline just inside the anus will ease the passage of the stool and thus relieve pain on defecation.

Mistletoe: Mr J. R. from Hertfordshire reports: 'After a hectic time preparing for Christmas my haemorrhoids returned. I recently read that the application of mistletoe was a suggested cure, so I thought why not. My local friendly florist was pleased to give me the berries waiting to be thrown away. After washing them and applying between two pieces of gauze I experienced wonderful relief and a complete cure. The moral is – have your haemorrhoids over Christmas.'

Restless Legs

Restless Legs Syndrome is an obscure affliction in which an unpleasant creeping sensation is felt deep within the bone and muscle. 'It feels as if my whole leg is full of small worms,' is how one sufferer describes it, and another 'as if ants are running up and down my bones.' Movement of the legs provide the only solace and sufferers find it impossible to keep still. This torture is psychological as well as physical. The creeping sensation may persist for hours at a time, keeping the tormented victim up till four or five in the morning and this forced insomnia unsettles the mind, inducing hallucinations and depression.

Medical examinations reveal no abnormality; nor do other investigatory tests. No abnormalities of muscles or nerves have ever been identified. The cause is unknown, though it is presumed there must be some area deep in the brain from which the crawling sensation originates.

Those who suffer from restless legs will get little help from their doctors who are as mystified by the complaint as they are, and for which they have no certain cure to offer. Several contributors have, however, suggested a variety of remedies which could be tried.

Heat: Heat in the form of a hot bath last thing at night or a hot water bottle and bed socks can prevent restless legs. Blessed relief is sometimes reported during a viral illness such as flu which, by raising the temperature, provides solace for a few days.

Cold: Alternatively, some sufferers find relief by pouring icy water over their legs, lying horizontal on the ground and sticking their feet in the refrigerator or, weather permitting, walking barefoot in the snow.

Exercise: 'Lie on the floor and "cycle" in the air until the muscles ease up.' Anon.

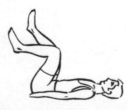

Cramp: Fascinatingly, deliberately inducing an attack of cramp can bring relief, as described by Mr J. I. Visser from Edinburgh.

> 'Having been driven up the wall (literally) with restless legs and tried everything, eventually out of desperation, I pulled my calf muscles so tight that very quickly I got cramp in the leg. Letting go, I immediately noticed the infernal irritation had just about disappeared. Now when I feel the restless legs are about to start up again, I induce a cramp, let go immediately and have no more trouble. Sometimes I have to repeat the process a few times but no more.'

There may be a further connection between restless legs and cramps because Mr U. G. Huggins from East Sussex reports that after being advised to drink 'lots of tonic water at night' as a home remedy for night cramps, 'I am glad to say that after two months the problem was almost completely solved'.

Water: Emeritus surgeon Mr T. P. N. Jenkins from Surrey reports he has been 'plagued by restless legs from my late teens into my eighties. It was a great event in my life when I discovered a simple solution – a drink of water. As the discomfort of restless legs impinges on sleep, a point is reached when it is well worthwhile to get out of bed and drink. In a few minutes, the symptoms ease off and a deep sleep returns'.

Sex Selection

Many couples nowadays having had two children of the same sex are keen to have another – but only if it is of the opposite sex. There is thus a natural interest in the question of whether in some way or another couples might be able to influence the sex of their offspring by sex selection. This can obviously be readily achieved by antenatal diagnosis which by determining the sex of the foetus makes it possible to selectively abort any of the 'wrong' sex. Such a practice is outlawed in Britain so couples must resort to other means for which, though they certainly sound ingenious, there is no serious evidence of their effectiveness.

The sex of children is determined by whether the ovum is fertilised by a sperm carrying the usual twenty-three chromosomes together with the female sex X chromosome, or twenty-three chromosomes together with the male sex Y chromosome. They are called X and Y because of their shape and the only physical difference between the two is that the Y chromosome is missing one arm's length, so the sperm carrying it is infinitesimally slightly less heavy. Clearly, if sex selection is to work, it is necessary to separate the two types of sperm, and there must be some other distinguishing physical characteristic that allows this to be done.

In 1970 Dr Landrum Shettles, an American gynaecologist, reported that the Y bearing sperm swims faster and so, other things being equal, they should get to the ovum first and many more boys than girls would be born. But this is balanced, he claimed, by the fact that the X bearing female sperm, though less speedy, are more resilient and so less likely to be destroyed by vaginal secretions which are more acidic around the crucial time of ovulation.

If this theory is correct then it is possible to practice do-it-yourself sex selection.

For a girl: Couples wishing to have a girl should first douche the vagina with a diluted teaspoonful of acidic white vinegar which will selectively 'knock off' the competing sperm carrying the male Y chromosome. In addition they should be sure to have sexual intercourse immediately around the time of ovulation – which can be determined by a slight rise in body temperature and the presence of a clear jelly-like vaginal discharge – as this gives the 'female' bearing sperm an equal chance against the male.

For a boy: By contrast, for those who wish to have a boy, the woman should douche the vagina with a diluted alkaline solution of sodium bicarbonate, thus rendering the environment less hostile to the male Y bearing sperm. In addition sexual activity should occur either just before or just after ovulation to maximise on the Y bearing sperm's ability to swim faster.

Dr Shettles subsequently proposed a further modification based on the observation that when the woman has an orgasm her vaginal secretions tend to be alkaline and so only those wishing to have a boy should try to achieve this pleasurable plateau.

Dr Shettles has sold a lot of books describing his techniques presumably because even if the method is completely valueless, half of all the couples following his advice would by chance end up with a child of their desired sex.

Skin Ulcers

Following an abrasion, a poorly healing wound on the legs due to poor circulation can be very slow to heal. Honey is the traditional remedy whose use was first recorded by the Egyptians in 2000 BC and as Mr P. J. Armon, consultant gynaecologist, reports continues to this day.

'Honey has been used in the treatment of infected wounds at the Kilimanjaro Medical Centre in Tanzania for the past four years with excellent results. In one case a woman was admitted with a massive post partum haemorrhage, requiring emergency hysterectomy and five further operations to deal with intestinal obstruction and abscesses. During the course of this debilitating illness she developed a massive bedsore on her sacrum, 15–20 centimetres in size, exposing the bone. The surface of the sore was covered three times daily with a thin layer of pure honey and a dry dressing. Twenty-one days later the cavity had closed without surgical treatment and the sacrum was covered in a new layer of skin. Only one seven-day course of antibiotics had been used during this time.'

Mrs Elaine Field from Cornwall records a similar if less dramatic result.

'I have had for six months or more flaky skin on the top joint of my ring finger. After being given some hydrocortisone ointment by the chemist I then had a huge weeping sore which my doctor thought might be cancerous and accordingly referred me to a specialist. In the meantime my finger looked so awful I had to cover the sore when I left the house and each time smeared honey over the patch. Within two weeks it was completely clear and has not returned. I consider honey a miracle cure.'

Snoring

The nearest most people come to murdering their partners or spouses is when they are woken yet again by stentorian snoring from the adjoining pillow. Snoring is no laughing matter; it can wreck relationships, disrupt families and indeed be harmful to health. A heavy snorer suffers from chronic exhaustion and is more prone to heart ailments.

Snoring occurs when the tissues at the back of the throat, in sleep, collapse inwards, so that inspired air has to pass through a very narrow aperture – producing the characteristic grunting sounds. In its most severe form the narrowing at the back of the throat can be so extreme that breathing may stop altogether – a condition known as obstructive sleep apnoea or OSA. A person with OSA is, as it were, suffering from self-strangulation – the oxygen concentration in the blood falls to a point where the breathing centre in the brain is stimulated to make another voluntary intake of breath.

Those with OSA get insufficient restful sleep – they wake with a headache in the morning, are sleepy during the day and fall asleep at the slightest opportunity, whether at work, in church or while driving a car and sometimes in the middle of a meal.

Heavy snoring is thus a potentially serious condition which needs proper medical evaluation, but there are several simple remedies, each working in a different way, that can alleviate or abolish snoring, thus obviating the need for more drastic remedies.

Cut down on alcohol: There is no harm in a couple of glasses of wine in the evening and even a night-cap, but serious drinking in the evening is a major contributory factor to snoring for two reasons: a lot of alcohol in the bloodstream at night reduces the body's movements when asleep while simultaneously suppressing the breathing centre in the brain. Thus the typical position of the hard drinking heavy snorer is of a person flat on his back emitting intermittent snoring grunts.

Snoring

Lose weight: This is, of course, easier said than done but reducing the amount of body fat all over will also reduce the quantity of tissues at the back of the throat and thus there is less to collapse inwards to obstruct the inflow of breath.

Steam: Nasal stuffiness is a potent cause of snoring by preventing breathing through the nose, forcing all the air that is inhaled and exhaled through the mouth. Hence those with a cold or hay fever tend to be heavy snorers, and it is only sensible to clear and open up the nasal passages at night by placing hot water in a flat pan, throwing a towel over the head and breathing in and out for ten minutes.

Marbles: Dr George McGeary from Oregon describes this interesting snoring cure. 'It was suggested by my mother who sewed a small glass marble into the pyjama top between the shoulder blades under a scrap of cloth. When the snorer rolls on his or her back, he immediately rolls back on his side usually without waking and resumes sleep without snoring. Once a marble is sewn into the pyjamas it can be forgotten about – as they go through the wash without problems.'

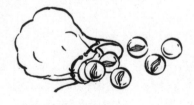

Dr Fritz Shmerl, a physician from California, has suggested a variant on this theme. 'I advise the use of half a soft sponge rubber ball six centimetres in diameter. Such a ball is available in any toy shop. Its hemisphere is detached and fastened to the mid part of the back of the pyjama top. I use friction material such as Velcro that when glued to the flat disc of the half ball clings firmly to the pyjamas fitted with a complementary piece.'

Cottonwool: The alternative to treating the snorer is to treat the partner. When the ears are plugged with cottonwool at night, the sounds of snoring become much fainter and sleep is no longer disturbed.

Sore Throat

Family doctors will, on average, see four patients with a sore throat each week. This adds up to around 150,000 consultations a year in Britain, for which they prescribe £22.5 million worth of antibiotics. This may be appropriate for a small minority where it is obviously a bacterial infection usually caused by the bug streptococcus. Here the back of the throat is grossly inflamed with signs of pus or an abscess, the throat glands are enlarged and painful, and the temperature is raised.

For most, however, the cause of the sore throat is a virus which does not respond to antibiotics and so will simply get better of its own accord. Here the best treatment is to control the main symptoms of pain and swelling and simple remedies, by avoiding the hazards of inappropriate antibiotics, are clearly useful. The particular efficacy of the 'cold cloth' cure – advocated by several contributors – is of particular interest as most people, including doctors, are unaware of it.

Salt and water gargle: Gargling with salt water, or an antiseptic such as TCP three or four times a day, will sterilise the back of the throat and promote healing of the inflamed tissues. It is perhaps less well appreciated that both soluble aspirin and spirits such as whisky or brandy have a local anaesthetic effect, so regular gargling with these remedies will reduce the pain associated with a sore throat.

Lemon juice and honey: This combination is an excellent remedy for sore throats where the astringent antiseptic properties of the lemon are offset by the soothing (and anti-infective) effects of the honey. They should be mixed together in hot water or tea and sipped throughout the day.

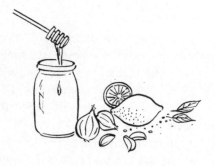

Cold cloth cure: One of my readers from Nottingham was brought up in Lancashire where her father was a chemist. The family lived on the shop premises so there was plenty of medical treatment on hand but nonetheless her mother's favourite remedy was the cold towel treatment. 'A large handkerchief was wrung out in cold water and laid around the neck and covered with a woollen scarf on retiring to bed. As far as I can remember it always worked.'

Mrs Margaret Bellord from Hertfordshire also testifies to this treatment pointing out in particular that the water has to be very cold – and as the cloth warms up, 'it was horribly uncomfortable . . . but it worked.'

Splinters

The conventional method of removing splinters – with a sterilised safety pin – causes some discomfort which can be avoided with the following remedy, suggested by Mrs Jane Morgan from Leigh on Sea.

> 'The solution to the removal of a splinter has been used in my family for many years successfully. You simply put some soft soap (from underneath the tablet which somebody always leaves floating in the bath) on a piece of lint. Add a small amount of brown sugar (it must be brown), place over the site of the splinter and stick down firmly with a plaster. Leave overnight and, hey presto, the splinter will be on the lint in the morning.'

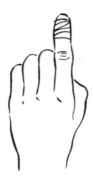

Independent confirmation of this striking remedy comes from Mrs Mary Rosewarne from Howe who tried it out on a splinter she had had in her finger for five days. 'The following morning, as I removed the plaster from my finger, the splinter actually started "rising" like a worm coming straight up out of the ground!'

Split Skin

Splitting of the skin causes painful fissures (collo-quially known as hacks) most often at the tips of the fingers or around the heel. There are several good proprietary preparations including Lotil and 'New Skin' which one contributor says should be 'painted over a whisp of cottonwool placed over the crack first.' Two other popular remedies are as follows:

Superglue: Mr J. C. Clarke, a retired anaesthetist from Belfast, reports that 'painful fissures can be instantly rendered painless by the use of Superglue. The fissures should be clean and dry. Carefully fill the open fissure with bubble-free Superglue and allow to dry. As healing takes place, the scab falls away spontaneously.' However, Mrs Mary Elliott from Essex was not so impressed. 'The Superglue certainly healed the crack but a few days later the skin around the thumb started to peel away all the way down to the first joint.' There is also the obvious danger of inadvertently sticking your fingers together – or to other things.

Sellotape: Mr David Fairburn from Argyle reports: 'I have suffered for many of my 68 years from "hacks". Some years ago in frustration I wound myself up in Sellotape – the hacks were completely cured in a matter of hours. Being quite unscientific I proceeded to treat some of the hacks with the tape and to leave others untreated. The untreated hacks remained for days but the treated ones cured without exception overnight.'

Stings

BEES, WASPS AND HORNETS

Bees, wasps and hornets inject their venom under the skin causing redness, swelling and pain which can last several hours unless prompt action is taken. The initial treatment of honey bee stings is different from others because they leave behind their barbed stinger embedded in the skin. This must be removed promptly to reduce the total amount of venom injected. Standard advice has been that the barb should be flicked off with a knife or other sharp object rather than pinched off as the latter procedure will increase the amount of venom injected.

This, it now appears, is not the case, for reasons outlined by Dr Kirk Visscher of the University of California. 'The advice that people should be concerned about how bee stings are removed is counter-productive. The method of removal is irrelevant, but even slight delays in removal caused by concern over the correct procedure, or finding an appropriate implement, are likely to increase the dose of venom received. The advice should simply be to emphasise that a bee sting should be removed as quickly as possible.'

Honey bee stings are of particular concern because they can attract other bees to sting the victim. Dr Visscher comments: 'The most important response to bees defending their nests should be to get away from the vicinity as quickly as possible. An alarm chemical is emitted at the base of the honey bee sting; when detected by other bees it helps them in localising the victim and making them more likely to sting. In such a situation, reaching safety is much more important than removing the sting immediately.'

By contrast it is recommended that the immediate response to a wasp sting should be to suck it out before the hole closes up. 'Father always said he could taste the bitterness if it was done in time. You should, of course, spit it out,' writes Mrs Marian Banyard from Suffolk.

Irrespective of the cause of the sting, the main priority is to reduce the pain, for which there are a variety of home remedies to choose from.

Cold: Ice cubes placed on the sting have a local anaesthetic effect, reduce the swelling and prevent he spread of the venom.

Heat: Heat in the form of a hot flannel or hairdryer directed at the sting may be equally effective.

Sodium Bicarbonate: A paste of water and sodium bicarbonate has a favourable soothing effect.

Mud: In the countryside without access to hot water or ice cubes, a paste of earth and water covered with a bandage is recommended.

Cigarettes: This is a variant of the heat remedy. Mr Eric Wardroper from the Dordogne area of France, whose wife is allergic to wasp stings, comments: 'The local people of this area always keep cigarettes and matches handy. When stung, light a cigarette and hold it as close to the sting as comfort allows. Keep it there until it has burnt the whole length. This stops the poison spreading and saves a lot of discomfort. We are non-smokers but always keep cigarettes in the medicine cabinet, the car and my wife's handbag for such an emergency.'

Scorpion Stings

Mrs T. M. Godber from Somerset reports the following remedy for scorpion stings from the time she lived in a rubber planter's bungalow in Malaya. 'My younger sister stood on a scorpion and was stung on the sole of the foot. It was New Year's Eve and we all thought she would be unable to enjoy the dance that evening to celebrate the occasion. Our Chinese cook volunteered a proven antidote. We crushed the scorpion and applied it to the wound, bandaging it in place. She had scarcely any swelling or discomfort and was able to enjoy the dance as planned.'

Stings in the Mouth or Throat

The danger with stings in the mouth is that they can cause the tissues to swell. The victim should suck on an ice cube or cold water and spit out. If there is the slightest sign of difficulty in breathing then prompt medical attention should be sought.

Stitch

The cause of the crippling pain in the upper abdomen usually on the right following exercise, commonly known as a stitch, is a medical mystery. It can be precipitated by eating a large meal but more frequently by exercise that jolts the body like running on hard ground or in boggy countryside. It is particularly common in horse (and even more so camel) riders but rare in swimmers, skaters and cyclists.

The most plausible theory is that a stitch is caused by stretching of the ligaments which hold the gut in place, and on these grounds the following remedies are proposed, firstly prevention and then treatment.

Prevention: No food or water should be taken for two to four hours before exercise. In addition, the abdominal muscles should be strengthened by lying down with raised knees and hips and raising the head towards the upper chest.

Treatment: Stand on your head.

Styes

A stye is caused by blockage of the hair follicle of an eyelash behind which a small collection of infected material accumulates. The usual medical treatment is with an antibiotic cream but there are a variety of remedies that are equally or more effective.

Hot compresses: Hot compresses are a reliable way of bringing the stye to a head. The simplest method is to apply to the eyelash cottonwool or a piece of gauze that has been dipped in hot water to which salt has been added.

Saliva: The anti-infective properties of saliva make it a suitable treatment for styes. Regular applications of early morning spittle to a stye in its early stages will prevent it developing.

Wedding ring: This remedy is particularly interesting because it illustrates so well the difference between the superstitious nonsense of the 'old wives tale' from the genuine article.

In *Country Things* by Alison Uttley, published in

1946, she writes 'to cure a stye, the eyelid is rubbed very gently with pure gold. A wedding ring is used for this without, of course, removing it from the finger which would be unlucky. It has to be drawn three times across the afflicted eye. My mother often touched somebody's stye with her ring and even the most obstinate one disappeared within a few hours.'

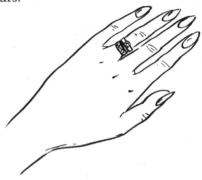

Mrs Mary Goodby from Chester puts the record straight about 'this excellent treatment'. 'In most homes mother's worn, plain gold wedding band is likely to be the only item in the house which is absolutely smooth without any possible points or corners, non-toxic, very clean due to mum's hands being constantly in water, and a convenient size for the job.'

The precise technique is as follows: 'Hold ring very firmly by its edge, between finger and thumb. Gently press the opposite half circle onto the affected eyelid whilst avoiding any possible pressure on the eyeball by performing a sort of gentle scooping action aiming under the stye itself. This causes the stye to empty of pus without hurting the inflamed part around the stye or the eye. An experienced mother could gently turn back the upper or lower eyelid and apply the ring just inside the edge of the lid.'

Thrush

Thrush is caused by a yeast – candida albicans – which commonly resides harmlessly in the vagina where it causes no symptoms. Factors that upset the delicate ecology of the vagina will result in the proliferation of the yeast, giving rise to the typical symptoms of itchiness and a white discharge. These include antibiotics taken for infections elsewhere in the body, hormones such as the contraceptive pill and HRT, or irritation of the vagina by tampons or insufficient lubrication at intercourse.

The antifungal preparation Canestan is an excellent cure for thrush and can be purchased readily over the counter from the chemist. This is much the best solution for the one-off attack. Those prone to recurrent episodes of thrush should consider the following remedies.

Salt and water: Much relief can be gained by adding a good handful of salt to a bidet or shallow bath and swishing around in the resulting brine.

Vinegar: Vinegar has a similar acidity to the vagina, which is believed to control the proliferation of the yeast. Vaginal acidity can be restored by douching in a mixture of four teaspoonfuls of vinegar to half a litre of warm water.

Hair dryer: Drying the vaginal area with a hairdryer rather than a towel will minimise irritation of the region.

Clothes: Warm and damp environments promote the growth of yeasts so it is advised that loose fitting cotton underwear should be worn close to the skin. Cutting the gusset out of tights promotes circulation of air to the genital area.

Live yoghurt: Live yoghurt contains the harmless bug lactobacillus and helps suppress the proliferation of candida in the vagina. It is advised that a pot of live yoghurt eaten every day will control the irritation and a small amount on the tip of a tampon can be introduced directly into the vagina.

Toothache

The cure for toothache is to take some painkillers, gargle with salty warm water and make an appointment to see the dentist as soon as possible. The following temporary remedy from Mr W. K. Ayres of Canterbury recalls the time when people were unable to afford to see the dentist and had no alternative other than to treat themselves.

'We lived in a small village seven miles from Dover. My father was a farmer renting his land. In those days there were no subsidies and he had two successive bad years. The first was a drought – some idiot of a boy set fire to a barn full of corn. By the time the horse-drawn fire brigade from a village two and a half miles away arrived there was nothing left. By direct contrast, in the summer of the next year we had a cloudburst over the village. So you can see we were not very well off and if we had toothache there was no chance of a visit to the dentist.

'My mother filled a large saucer with vinegar, sprinkled a good amount of pepper on it and soaked a square brown paper on it. When it was thoroughly wet she slapped it on the cheek nearest the offending tooth and tied it with a large handkerchief. I think it helped because we always slept quite well but it didn't pay to wriggle one's face in the pillow because the vinegar had evaporated and the brown paper felt like sandpaper.'

This brown paper and vinegar, of course, features as a remedy for another ailment – Jack's headache after 'breaking his crown' in the children's nursery rhyme Jack and Jill.

Warts

Warts can occur virtually anywhere in the body but most commonly on the hands and fingers where they are unaesthetic, and on the feet (known as verrucas) where they can be painful. They are caused by a virus – the human papilloma virus – and can spread from one site of the body to another. They are probably only slightly infective so difficult to 'catch' from someone else, though it is commonly believed that verrucas may be acquired from communal swimming baths.

The only interesting thing about warts is how to get rid of them and here there are essentially two standard options. The first is to obtain from the chemist (or doctor on prescription) a paint or gel which contains salicyclic acid which when regularly applied over a period of three months usually manages to eradicate them. The suggested technique is first to soak the wart in warm water for a couple of minutes, dry it and then carefully apply the paint and allow it to dry. This produces an elastic film over the wart which should be carefully removed and the procedure repeated the following day. The surface of the wart should then be rubbed with a pumice stone or piece of sand paper once a week.

The second standard therapy is to burn the warts off with liquid nitrogen which acts much more quickly. This treatment is usually only performed by skin specialists in the local hospital for which there is usually a waiting list of three months before being seen. So either way it takes quite a time to get rid of the wart – time enough to try one of several simple remedies.

More than any of the other remedies described in this book, those for warts are probably the least convincing and most vulnerable to the charge 'quackery'. Their efficacy is very difficult to assess because most – perhaps 75 per cent – of warts could disappear of their own accord without any treatment within a couple of years.

Many of the remedies are indeed 'quackery', such as the advice that the wart should be rubbed with a piece of meat which should be buried 'secretly', or the advice to wash the wart in the light of the moon. Nonetheless, despite their superstitious nature, such remedies could still work as warts are one of those human conditions that are wholly amenable to suggestion – that is, if the person believes strongly enough in the remedy, the warts will indeed disappear.

Thus, Dr Christopher McEwen, skin specialist from Louisiana reports: 'I have treated a couple of children who could not tolerate freezing (with liquid nitrogen). So I gave them a harmless substance to use and impressed upon them it was a very strong medicine that would knock out the warts. And it worked.'

In a similar vein Dr Nicholas Spanos, psychologist from Ottawa, described the effect of encouraging wart sufferers to spirit their warts away with visual imagery. 'We tell patients to imagine their warts are shrinking, that they can feel the tingling as their warts dissolve and their skin becomes clear. Those who report really vivid imagery are more likely to lose their warts than those who say their imagery was weak.'

The most frequently recommended of the many suggested home remedies for warts include the following:

Saliva: Saliva has anti-infective properties which may be effective against the papilloma virus. 'My method is to apply saliva to the offending spot. I first discovered the remedy by nibbling away at a wart on the knuckle of one of my fingers. Warts outside the nibbling range have to be dealt with by wetting the tip of the finger and applying the saliva in that manner.' Mr K. S. M. Sears from Surbiton.

Several contributors report that the best effects are obtained with saliva obtained first thing in the morning – 'fasting spittle'.

Broad bean pods: 'Some years ago I had a verruca which persisted for over two years despite the best efforts of my doctor and the fact that I had developed a slight limp. When listening to the radio one day I heard a man saying he had been similarly afflicted and his doctor had advised him to use broad bean pods rubbed on night and morning. I immediately started doing this – it being the right season for broad beans – and within three weeks the verruca disappeared never to return.' Mrs V. Haslam from Kent. A variant of this broad bean cure is to use the inside of a banana skin.

Dettol: 'A cure for verrucas that has never once failed in the thirty-six years I have been recommending it, is to soak the foot each night in water as hot as you can bear it then dab with undiluted

Dettol. The verruca dropped out in a week.' Mr W. Cassel from Sittingbourne.

Suggestion: Sometimes suggestion works and sometimes it does not. Mr R. E. Paul from Oxfordshire recalls:

> 'As a small boy in the twenties my hands were covered with warts which my mother was convinced were caused by my handling of milk churns on a farm where we frequently helped with the milking. Conventional treatment, mainly burning with a caustic pencil, had only limited success so another country remedy was tried. My mother gave me a small piece of steak and instructed me to rub this on the warts and bury the steak in the garden at night revealing to no one the site of the internment. This treatment also failed and on the advice of a neighbour, mother then took me to see a local countryman who was known as a wart charmer. The old gentleman consulted his calendar and asked me to come back on a certain date, the night of the full moon. On the appointed night I presented myself apprehensively and was taken out into the garden where Mr Hunt took my hands in his and fingered all the warts while gazing up at the moon and muttering some inaudible implication. He then said to me "Don't thank me and don't pay me or else the charm will not work." I did not believe this rigmarole for a minute but within a few days, all the warts had completely disappeared never to return.'

Wind

Trapped wind in the colon can cause abdominal discomfort and distension. Charcoal tablets, available from the chemist, can by absorbing excess gas, provide short term relief. The best method of dispersing trapped wind was discovered by accident by a patient admitted to hospital with toxic megacolon – an inflammatory condition of the bowel which becomes grossly distended with vast quantities of gas.

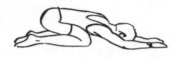

While trying to make himself more comfortable, the patient adopted the Mecca position – kneeling on the bed bent forward with his arms stretched out in front and his bottom sticking up in the air. In this position he passed a quantity of flatus 'which continued for several minutes'. He immediately felt more comfortable so he repeated this manoeuvre several times 'with similar results'. He described his experience to his astonished surgeon, Mr M. Z. Panos of the University of Birmingham, who measured his abdominal girth and discovered he had indeed become a lot slimmer. 'Over the next fortnight his condition gradually improved at which point he was discharged fully recovered,' comments Dr Panos.

It has subsequently become standard practice for surgeons to prescribe the 'Mecca position' in such circumstances, thus avoiding much unnecessary surgery. The same technique is also likely to be of value for those with trapped or excess wind for other reasons such as constipation or an over-consumption of beans.

References

Introduction

1 J. H. Marks, 'Chewing gum and eyelashes', *Journal of the American Medical Association*, Feb. 25, 1961, p. 740.
2 Graham Worrall, 'Acyclovir in recurrent herpes labialis', *British Medical Journal* (1996), vol. 313, p. 6.
3 Paul Addison, *Now the War is Over* (Jonathan Cape, 1985).

The Evidence

1 Svante Travenius, 'Alcohol and herpes labialis', *New Scientist*, Sept. 14, 1996, p. 53.
2 Mary Stone, 'Bactericidal activity of wet cerumen', *Ann. Otol. Rhinol. Laryngol.* (1984), pp. 93, 183–6.

Water

1 David Tyrrell et al, 'Local hyperthermia benefits natural and experimental common colds', *BMJ* (1989), vol. 298, pp. 1280–3.
2 Michael L. Macknin et al, 'Effects of inhaling heated vapour on symptoms of the common cold', *Journal of the American Medical Association* (1990), vol. 264, pp. 989–91.
3 Dov Ophir and Yigal Elad, 'Effects of steam inhalation on nasal patency and nasal symptoms in patients with a common cold', *American Journal of Otolaryngology* (1987), vol. 3, pp. 149–53.
4 Adrian W. Zorgniotti et al, 'Chronic scrotal hypothermia: results in 90 infertile couples', *Journal of Urology* (1985), vol. 135, pp. 944–47.

Alcohol

1 Jack Pickleman, 'A glass a day keeps the doctor . . .', *The American Surgeon* (1990), vol. 56, pp. 395–7.
2 R. S. Illingworth, 'Infantile colic revisited', *Archives of Disease in Childhood* (1985), vol. 60, pp. 981–5.
3 Martin E. Weisse et al, 'Wine as a digestive aid: comparative antimicrobial effect of bismuth salicylate

References

and red and white wine', *BMJ* (1995), vol. 311, pp. 1657–60.

Honey

1 David Greenwood, 'Honey for superficial wounds and ulcers', *The Lancet* (1993), vol. 341, p. 90.

2 A. Zumla and A. Luat, 'Honey – a remedy rediscovered', *Journal of the Royal Society of Medicine* (1989), vol. 82, p. 384.

3 Robert Blomfield, 'Honey for decubitus ulcers', *Journal of the American Medical Association* (1987), vol. 224, p. 905.

4 M. Subrahmanyam, 'Topical application of honey in treatment of burns', *British Journal of Surgery* (1991), vol. 78, pp. 497–8.

5 I. E. Haffejee, 'Honey in the treatment of infantile gastroenteritis', *BMJ* (1985), vol. 290, pp. 1866–7.

Sugar

1 B. Bose. 'Honey or sugar in treatment of infected wounds?', *The Lancet* (1982), I. p. 963.

2 R. Chirife et al, 'Scientific basis for use of granulated sugar in treatment of infected wounds', *The Lancet* (1982), I. p. 560.

3 H. Gordon, K. Middleton et al, 'Sugar and wound healing', *The Lancet* (1985), II. pp. 663–4.

4 L. A. Ramenghi et al, 'Effect of non-sucrose sweet tasting solutions on neonatal heal prick responses', *Archives of Disease in Childhood* (1996), vol. 74, pp. 129–31.

Yoghurt

1 Beverley A. Friend & Khem Shahani, 'Nutritional and therapeutic aspects of lactobacilli', *Journal of Applied Nutrition* (1984), vol. 36, pp. 125–53.

2 Victor Bokkenheuser, 'The friendly anaerobes', *Clinical Infectious Diseases* (1993), vol. 16 (suppl. 4), S427–34.

Chicken Soup

1 K. Saketkhoo et al, 'Effects of drinking hot water, cold water and chicken soup on nasal mucous velocity and nasal airflow resistance', *Chest* (1978), vol. 74, pp. 408–10.

2 David H. Spodick et al, 'The chicken soup contro-versy', *Chest* (1975), vol. 68, pp. 604–6.

3 Fred Rosner, 'Hot chicken soup for asthma, *The Lancet* (1979), II. p. 1079.

Fruit Juice

1 A. E. Sobota, 'Inhibition of bacterial adherence by cranberry juice: potential use for the treatment of urinary tract infections', *Journal of Urology* (1984), vol. 131, pp. 1013–15.

2 Harriet D. Khan et al, 'Effect of cranberry juice on urine', *Journal of the American Dietetic Association* (1967), vol. 51, pp. 251–4.

Tea and Coffee

1 P. C. Cheo and R. C. Lindner, 'In vitro and in vivo effects of commercial tannic acid on tobacco mosaic virus', *Virology* (1964), vol. 24, pp. 414–25.

2 Shmuel Kivity et al, 'The effect of caffeine on exer-cise-induced bronchoconstriction, *Chest* (1990), vol. 97, pp. 1083–5.

3 J. C. Henderson et al, 'Decrease of histamine-induced bronchoconstriction by caffeine in mild asthma', *Thorax* (1993), vol. 48, pp. 824–6.

Saliva

1 F. Lagerlof and A. Oliveby, 'Caries – protective factors in saliva', *Advances in Dental Research*. (1994), vol. 8, pp. 229–35.

2 Frank A. Scannapieco, 'Saliva–bacterium inter-actions in oral microbial ecology', *Critical Reviews in Oral Biology and Medicine* (1994), vol. 5, pp. 203–48.

3 W. M. Edgar, 'Saliva: its secretion, composition and functions', *British Dental Journal*, April 25, 1992, pp. 305–12.

Earwax

1 S. Megarry et al, 'The activity against yeasts of human cerumen', *Journal of Laryngology and Otology* (1988), vol. 102, pp. 671–2.

2 Isabelle Okuda, 'The organic composition of earwax', *Journal of Otolaryngology* (1991), vol. 20, pp. 212–5.

References

3 Mary Stone, 'Bactericidal activity of wet cerumen', *Ann. Otol. Rhinol. Laryngol.* (1984), vol. 93, pp. 183–5.

Urine
1 Coen van der Kroen, *The Complete Guide to Urine Therapy* (Amethyst Books, 1995).
2 Homer Smith, 'De Urina', *Journal of the American Medical Association* (1994), vol. 155, pp. 899–902.
3 J. U. Schlegel, 'Bactericidal affect of urea', *Journal of Urology* (1961), vol. 86, pp. 819–22.
4 Leon Muldavin, 'Treatment of infected wounds with urea', *The Lancet* (1938), I. pp. 549–51.
5 K. B. Bjornesjo, 'Tuberculostatic factor in normal human urine', *American Review of Tuberculosis* (1956), vol. 73, p. 967.

Individual entries:

Arthritis
1 Janet Cudshnaghan et al, 'Taping the patella medially: a new treatment for osteoarthritis of the knee joint?', *BMJ* (1994), vol. 308, pp. 753–5.
2 Dava Sobel and Arthur C. Klein, *Arthritis: What Really Works* (Robinson 1994).

Athlete's Foot
1 John M. B. Smith, 'Interdigital athlete's foot: the battle for survival occurring between our toes', *New Zealand Medical Journal*, October 26, 1983, pp. 799–800.
2 Colin Ryall, 'The ecology of athlete's foot', *New Scientist*, Aug. 14, 1980, pp. 528–30.

Boils
1 Jill Nice, *Herbal Remedies and Home Comforts* (Piatkus, 1990).

Breast Feeding
1 V. Cheryl Nikodem et al, 'Do cabbage leaves prevent breast engorgement? A randomised, controlled study', *Birth* (1993), vol. 20, pp. 61–4.

Broken Rib
1 K. Norcross, 'Strapping up the broken rib', *The Lancet* (1980), I. pp. 589–90.

Choking
1 W. C. Eller and R. K. Haugen, 'Food asphyxiation – restaurant rescue', *New England Journal of Medicine*, July 12, 1973, pp. 81–2.
2 Editorial, 'Death at the dining table: a fallible diagnosis', *The Lancet* (1973), II. p. 367.
3 Henry J. Heimlich, 'A lifesaving manoeuvre to prevent food choking', *Journal of the American Medical Association* (1975), vol. 234, pp. 398–401.
4 M. Dover 'Removing an obstruction from your own airway', *BMJ* (1996), vol. 312, p. 450.

Conjunctivitis
1 Coen van der Kroon, *The Complete Guide to Urine Therapy* (Amethyst Books, 1995).

Constipation
1 Jean Carper, *The Food Pharmacy* (Simon and Schuster, 1988).
2 D. P. Burkitt and H. C. Trowell, *Refined Carbohydrate Foods and Disease* (London, 1975), p. 65.

Deafness
1 J. F. Sharp et al, 'Earwax removal: a survey of current practice', *BMJ* (1990), vol. 301, pp. 1251–2.
2 Maurice Ernest, 'On the use of a plastic ketchup bottle as an aural syringe', *The Journal of Otolaryngology* (1991), vol. 20, p. 69.

Eyestrain
1 Jill Nice, *Herbal Remedies and Home Comforts* (Piatkus, 1990).

Foreign Bodies
1 Mason P. Thompson, 'Removing objects from the external auditory canal', *New England Journal of Medicine* (1984), vol. 311, p. 1635.
2 K. O'Toole et al, 'Removing cockroaches from the

References

auditory canal: controlled trial', *New England Journal of Medicine* (1985), vol. 312, p. 1197.
3 Eugene Guazzo, 'Removal of foreign bodies from the nose', *New England Journal of Medicine* (1985), vol. 312, p. 725.

Heartburn

1 Octavio Bessa, 'Tights pants syndrome – a new title for an old problem', *Archives Internal Medicine* (1993), vol. 153, p. 1396.

Hiccoughs

1 James Lewis, 'Hiccoughs: causes and cures', *Journal of Clinical Gastroenterology* (1985), vol. 7, pp. 539–52.
2 Francis Fesmire, 'Termination of intractable hiccoughs with digital rectal massage', *Annals of Emergency Medicine* (1988), vol. 17, p. 160.

Infant Colic

1 R. S. I. Illingworth, 'Infant Colic', *Archives of Disease in Childhood* (1985), vol. 60, pp. 981–5.

Infertility

1 Mark V. Sauer, 'Effects of abstinence on sperm motility in normal men,' *American Journal Obstetrics and Gynaecology* (1988), vol. 158, pp. 604–7.
2 Robert M. Levin et al, 'Correlation of sperm count with frequency of ejaculation', *Fertility and Sterility* (1986), vol. 45, pp. 732–5.
3 Adrian W. Zorgniotti et al, 'Chronic scrotal hypthermia: results in 90 infertile couples', *Journal of Urology* (1986), vol. 125, pp. 944–8.

Insomnia

1 Colin Espie, 'Practical management of insomnia: behavioural and cognitive techniques', *ABC of Sleep Disorders* (BMA Publications).

Nose Bleeds

1 Philip Turner, 'The swimmer nose clip in epistaxis', *J. Accid. Emerg. Med.*, (1996), vol. 13, p. 134.

Sex Selection
1 Kaye Wellings, 'Sex selection', *Which Way to Health?* April, 1993, pp. 49–51.
2 Robert H. Glass, 'Sex pre-selection', *Obstetrics & Gynaecology* (1977), vol. 49, pp. 122–6.

Skin Ulcers
1 P. J. Armon, 'The use of honey in the treatment of infected wounds', *Tropical Doctor*, April, 1980, p. 91.

Snoring
1 Sheila Jennett, 'Snoring and its treatment', *BMJ* (1984), vol. 289, pp. 335–6.
2 R. Michael Lattey, 'Simple solution to snoring', *Canadian Medical Association Journal* (1988), vol. 139, p. 286.
3 David Fairbanks, 'Non surgical treatment of snoring', *Otolaryngology Head and Neck Surgery* (1989), vol. 100, p. 233.
4 George McGeary and Fritz Schmerl, 'Help a snorer', *Journal of the American Medical Association* (1981), vol. 245, pp. 1729–30.

Sore Throat
1 H. Marcovitch, 'Sore throats', *Archives of Disease in Childhood* (1990), vol. 65, pp. 249–50.
2 John Pitts, 'What influences doctors prescribing? Sore throats revisted.' *Journal of the Royal College of General Practitioners*, Feb, 1989, pp. 65–6

Stings
1 P. K. Visscher et al, 'Removing bee stings', *The Lancet* (1996), vol. 348, pp. 301–2.

Stitch
1 J. D. Sinclair, 'Stitch: the side pain of athletes', *New Zealand Medical Journal* (1951), vol. 50, pp. 607–12.
2 Finn Rost, 'The stitch: the side pain of athletes', *New Zealand Medical Journal*, June 25, 1986, p. 469.

References

Warts
1 W. R. Bett, 'Wart, I bid thee be gone', *The Practitioner* (1951), vol. 166, pp. 77–80.
2 Alan M. Massing et al, 'Natural history of warts', *Archives of Dermatology* (1963), vol. 87, pp. 306–10.
3 C. McEwen and N. Spanos, in *The Doctors' Book of Home Remedies* (Rodale Health Books, 1994).

Wind
1 M. Z. Panos et al, 'Toxic megacolon: the knee-elbow position relieves bowel distension', *Gut* (1993), vol. 34, pp. 1726–7.

Acknowledgements

This book could not have been written without the help of many readers of the *Daily Telegraph*. They include:

Mr J. Aaron, Mr G. D. Adams, Mrs Ann Ainsworth, Mr H. J. Allen, Mr W. S. Annable, Mrs P. M. Ansell, Mrs Elizabeth Ardill, Ms P. Austin, Mrs Peggy Auton, Mr W. K. Ayers, Mr Ron Ayerst, Mr John Bainbridge, Mr A. L. Baker, Mr F. Baley, Mrs Marion Banyard, Miss M. D. Barnes, Mrs J. Barton, Mr John Bassett, Mr J. C. Beard, Mr Geoffrey Bellis, Mrs Margaret Bellord, Mr Edward Bennett, Mrs Constance Benton, Mrs Pamela Betts, Mrs Ann Birks, Mrs Daphne Blacock, W. D. Blake, Mrs Bet Bolt, Mrs Vivien Bolton, Mrs Hilary Bonye, Mrs P. R. Booth, Mr Derek Boxall, Mirja Boyd, Mrs Angela Breckon, A. C. J. Brent-Good, Mr Norman Bromley, Irene Broughton, Mr Ernest Brown, Mr John Brown, Mrs Nancy Brown, Mrs Julie Buchanan, Mrs Penny Bullivant, Mrs J. L. Butler, N. W. Byrne, Mrs M. D. Cameron, Margaret Cameron, Mr John Campbell, Mrs Evelyn Careless, Miss M. E. Caryfield, Mrs P. M. Caseley, Mr W. Cassel, Mrs Cynthia Castellan, Mr Robert Cawley, B. M. Charratt, Mrs Constance Clark, Mavis Clark, Miss R. T. Clark, Carolyn Clarke, Dr J. C. Clarke, Vera Clarke, Mrs Anne Claxton, Commander R. H. Colby RN, Mr Roy Collins, Mrs Helen Cooper, Colonel V. J. C. Cooper, Mrs S. Cortis, Mrs Mirren Coxon, G. W. J. Crawford, Mrs Sally Crinean, Mrs Christine Crosland, Mrs Barbara Daniels, Mrs I. E. Darnel, Professor D. A. M. Davies, J. H. Davies, Roberta Davies, Louise Dawson, Mrs Shirley De Ath, Mrs Julie De Vile, Mrs Margaret Dent, J. Derlien, Mrs Drummond Crabbe, Mr W. I. Drysdale, Mrs Irene Duncan, Mrs E. Eardill, Margaret Edy, Ms Mary Elliott, Mrs D. M. Evans, Mrs Irene Evans, Mr Brian Evers, Mr John Eyton-Jones, Mr Alan Fenemore, Mr David Fairburn, Mr P. J. Fenerty, Mrs Elaine Field, J. H. Fisher, Mrs Mary Flint, Miss Marie Flower, Lady Ford, Mrs Pat Franklin, Mr Derek Fraylen, D. Fryer, Miss B. J. Gadd,

Acknowledgements

Mr Norman Gardiner, Mrs M. S. Geering, Mrs F. A. B. George, Mr John Gilbert, Mrs T. M. Godber, Mrs D. P. Gomez, R. A. Goodbar, Mrs Mary Goodby, Mrs S. R. Goodman, Mrs Irene Goodrerd, Mr Paul Goriup, Mr Basil Gotto, Mr Alan Grant, Mr John Granville, M. Gray, Mr Cyril Green, Mr John Green, G. Green, Mr S. J. Green, Mr S. Greening-Jackson, Joan Greenup, Margaret Griffin, Mrs K. D. Hall, Mrs Margareta Hallam, A. G. Halligey, Professor J. M. T. Hamilton-Miller, Mr James Hannay, Miss M. L. B. Harberd, Florence Harrson, Mrs V. Haslam, Dorothy Hedley, Mrs Pauline Hemsley, C. Hepworth, Mrs P. Hester, Mrs V. J. B. Hibbert, Mrs M. Hill, Mrs David Hilton, Mr Robert Hilton, Mrs Geraldine Hobson, J. Hockley, Mrs J. Holland, Mrs E. C. Hood, Mr U. G. Huggins, A. W. Hutchinson, H. H. F. Hutchinson, Mrs Anne Irwin, Miss Barbara Ivy, Mr Morrison James, Mr T. P. N. Jenkins, Sheila Jennings, Mr R. D. Jephcott, Mr Stephen Jessop, Mrs Elise Johnston, Mrs Ruby Johnston, Mr J. Jolley, G. A. Jolly, Mrs Elizabeth Jones, Mrs Jill Jones, Mrs M. L. Jones, Mrs Diana Joslin, Irene Katchourin, Mr Michael Keef, Mr Niall Kennedy, Thea Kennedy, Mr W. T. Kermode, Mrs Ruth Kershaw, Mrs Sheila Kewlil, Mrs Mary King, Mrs N. M. King, Mrs E. M. Kirby, Margaret Kirtz, Mrs Jill Leaberry, Helen Lee, Gabriel Lewis, Mr Rory Linden-Kelly, Mr Alan Lord, Mr Roy Lowe, Angela Lyle, Miss Eileen Lynch, Mrs Kathleen Macdonald, Patricia MacLaren-Butler, Angela Maclean, Mrs Margaret Malloy, Mrs Edna Markiewicz, Mrs E. M. Martin, Mr John Maslen, Mr P. Mason, Lt Col H. P. S. Massy, Mr Matthews, Mrs Jill McAnee, Mrs Stella McCandless, Belinda Mead, Mr Douglas Meaden, Mrs Jill Mendel, Mrs Daphne Meryon, Mrs Barbara Middleton, Mr Peter Miles, Dr R. M. Miller, Mr Clive Mills, Brenda Mold, Mr Alastair Monroe, Mrs Jane Morgan, Mr J. Morley, Mrs H. M. Morrish, Mrs F. A. Murphy, Rowena Nesbitt, Mr Jeremy Nichols, Mr M. Nichols, J. A. Nicol, Mrs I. Northfield, Miss Patricia O'Driscoll, Sheila O'Reilly, Mr E. Oliver, Mrs Pamela Orpen, Mr H. Orr, Ms J. Orritt, Mr Jack Palmer, Mr T. W. Palmer, Mr Peter Parr, Mrs Mary Parsons, Mr John S. Paterson, Dr M. F. Paterson, Mr R. E. Paul, Miss Jean

A. Peale, Mr T. R. Pearce, Mr Clifton Pender, Mr G. L. Phillipson, Mrs Dinah Pichersfill, Mrs Joanne Pierce, Mrs G. S. Pink, Mrs Belinda Platt, Miss A. Powell, Mr G. V. Pride, Dr T. R. F. Raw, Mrs E. Redgrave, Mr Tom Rees-Jones, Evelyn Rice, Mr D. J. Richards, W. Robins, Miss Edith Rolfe, Jean Rooney, Mrs Mary Rosewarne, Mr H. Row, Peggy Rowell, Mr F. W. Sanders, Mr B. R. Sandwell, Mr K. S. M. Sears, F. Seiflow, Mrs P. Sherwood, Mr P. G. Shingler, Mrs Ellene Simmonds, D. J. Simpson, Mr S. A. Skinner, Mrs Jean Slater, Mrs Angela Smith, Dr John Smith, Mr K. E. Smith, Mrs K. R. Smith, M. D. Smith, Mrs R. J. Stanbury, Mrs Mary Stay, Mr J. Stewart, Mr Paul Stickley, Mr Andrew Stronach, Mr David Strudwick, Mrs A. J. Swaine, Thelma Swales, Mrs J. N. Swinscow, Mrs E. M. Tanfield, C. Tarleton, Mrs E. Taylor, Mrs Frances Taylor, R. C. N. Thomas, Mrs Marianne Ticehurst, S. J. Tims, Mr Paul Tunbridge, Mrs Sylva Usher, Janet Valentine, Mr J. I. Visser, Isobel Wagg, Dr E. S. Waight, A. Warburton, Mr E. O. Wardroper, G. T. Warner, Margaret Watson, Mrs D. Watt, Mr Chris Webb, Mrs Marjorie Wells, Mrs P. Whetton, Mrs A. White, Mrs M. E. Whitehead, Kathleen Whiteman, Mrs Margaret Wilkins, Mrs E. Wilkinson, Mr Martin Willcocks, Mrs Barbara Willett, Mrs Kathleen Williams, Mrs Linda Williams, Mr Allan Wilson, Eileen Wilson, Yvonne Wilson, Mrs Vivien Womersely, Mrs Marguerite Wood, Shelagh Wood, Mrs Evelyn Woodfield, Miss I. E. Woolford, Mrs Rosemary Wray, Lady Patsy Yardley, Mrs Gogi Younger, Mrs Joan Zetterholm.

Index

Index

Index

Index

Index